The
KETOGENIC DIET
For Athletes

The Ultimate Guide to Improving Athletic Performance

Charlotte Cambell

THIS BOOK IS DEDICATED TO MY PARENTS,
WITHOUT WHOSE LOVE AND SUPPORT I COULD
NOT HAVE WRITTEN THIS BOOK

TABLE OF CONTENTS

The ketogenic diet is gaining increasing attention in both the mainstream consciousness and the scientific, medical and athletic populations. There is a plethora of studies and research proclaiming the benefits and protocols and rightly so as our "health" as a Western civilisation is getting worse. Something has to change.

The incidence of chronic disease (stroke, heart disease and diabetes) is growing rapidly throughout Western civilisations and obesity rates are at epidemic proportions.

However, this book will not focus on targeting global disease and obesity as it is beyond the scope of our discussion and there are plenty of excellent books[1, 16,17] on this topic. Rather the focus here will be on how the ketogenic diet can apply to the health and performance of endurance athletes.

In endurance sports, what you eat in training is a huge issue in how well you can train and how quickly you recover. Also, on race day, what you eat and drink can see you producing the performance of your life or can put you out of the race completely if you get it wrong.

That being said, similar global health phenomena apply to athletes as well. There are many athletes who continue to get fatter despite large training volumes.

ATHLETES ARE OFTEN VERY FIT
BUT NOT ALWAYS VERY HEALTHY

Athletes can also have the dangerous tendency to think they are "invincible" as they are generally stronger and fitter than their peers. Athletes also develop their fair share of diabetes, heart disease and chronic illness despite being from a group who are "interested in looking after themselves".

But do they look after themselves?

Many athletes actually have a terrible diet because "they can get away with it"!

They may eat sugary drinks and junk food in large quantities "without putting on weight". This may be ok in the short term.

But in the long term, you cannot "out-train" a bad diet.

YOU CANNOT "OUT-TRAIN" A BAD DIET

If you want to be lean and healthy plus improve your athletic performance, your diet (your fuel) needs to be addressed and optimized.

It is not as simple as the calories in/calories out ratio to maintain a healthy weight and good health as many triathletes and marathon runners can attest to.

Despite exercising 20-30 hours a week for decades, many runners and triathletes are still fat and many continue to get fatter every year.

There is also a very high incidence of tooth decay and gum disease in athletic populations[39]! Think about it, if you require sugary sports drinks and gels every training session twice a day, that is a lot of sugar coating your teeth every day.

That is also a lot of insulin spikes throughout the day and high blood sugar levels the body has to process.

One solution to addressing this insidious ill-health and growing obesity problem lies not in calorie counting but in changing the quality of the calorie. *What* you eat matters far more than *how much* you eat. What you eat affects your hormones, which affects your fat accumulation.

THE BIGGEST CULPRIT IS INSULIN

When insulin levels are raised, you accumulate fat. When insulin drops, your body liberates fat and burns it for fuel.

Insulin production is stimulated by carbohydrate-rich foods, refined carbohydrates, starchy vegetables and sugars including sucrose and fructose[16].

If you can address this chronic stimulation of insulin, fat loss will become a lot easier.

What If I Am A Runner, Cyclist Or Triathlete?

Much of the research on the ketogenic diet is done on sedentary populations or on disease populations like cancer studies, diabetes studies and epilepsy studies. The results in these populations have been astounding and very encouraging.

However, I wanted to focus here on the needs of the endurance athletic population. We have different requirements than the general population. We generally require more calories than the standard 1500-2000 calories per day of sedentary office workers and we need a reliable source of extra energy over several hours of intense exercise.

One of the most common questions and concerns from triathletes and other endurance athletes is:

"How can I maintain enough energy for my sport and reduce the risk of stomach issues from ingesting too many sports gels?"

I wrote this book as I dug deeper for myself to find out how I could use the principles of this amazing diet to help endurance athletes. Information on the ketogenic diet for endurance athletes was a little sparse and tended to be spread out across multiple books, websites and studies. I wanted to bring it together into one place as a useful resource.

The main focus of this book is on endurance sports as the majority of you will be triathletes or endurance athletes.

If you are a triathlete or are thinking of trying a triathlon, you are welcome to join our Free 5-Day Triathlon Accelerator Course.

The Current Standard American Diet (SAD) And The Typical Athlete's Diet

In its simplest form, the purpose of food is to give us energy. Many scientists and athletes have been studying different diets for years to try to give them an "edge" whether that is:

- A business person who has more energy to work longer hours and think more clearly

  Or

- An athlete who can train harder and perform better as everyone else fatigues

Even though there is not one clear agreed on diet, what is now very clear is that the traditional food pyramid (the Standard American Diet) put out by Western governments now appears to be outdated, harmful and responsible for a significant increase in obesity and chronic disease.

The American Diet

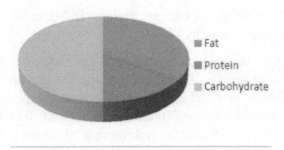

CARBOHYDRATE 50-60%

PROTEIN: 20%

FAT: 15-20%

The traditional food pyramid suggests getting 60% of your fuel from carbohydrate sources like breads, pasta, and rice. (Most people also include an insane amount of cookies, biscuits, cakes and sweets as well.)

This high intake of grains and sugars stimulates excess insulin production leading to lifelong insidious weight gain, chronic inflammation and elevated disease risk factors for auto-immune diseases, diabetes, cancers and heart disease.

This goes for athletes as well. Athletes have been taught to eat the usual 50-60% carbohydrate diet plus carbo-load on top of that prior to and during long events and races.

Athletes have been excessively marketed to for decades to stock up on gels, energy bars and carbo-rich sugary drinks and most of us do exactly this (thinking we are doing the right thing).

If you take a look around the developed world, there are record numbers of people suffering diabetes, cancers, heart disease and chronic illness—like gut disorders, obesity,

IBS and auto-immune disease.

Clearly whatever we are eating, as a rule, it is not working.

Something needs to change. Being "fit" does not always mean you are "healthy".

If you look around many athletic populations, many of the participants are still not in good shape. At the start line of any big city marathon, when you look at the participants, approximately 50% of them are fat. And this is after training for over 6 months and running 10-20 hours a week.

How is it possible to train hard 10-20 hours a week and still carry a spare tyre?

Sadly, many great athletes become disease ridden in their 40s and 50s with diabetes, heart problems, accelerated ageing and are often crippled with arthritis.

How can this be?

Our generation has so much information available at our fingertips that there is almost no excuse not to be at optimum health.

However, when we look around the incidence of chronic disease, it is through the roof. We are literally killing ourselves with food.

For me, I know that I want to perform well in my running, cycling, and swimming performances now. But I do not want to do this at the *expense* of my health, rather I am looking to enhance my athletic performance *and* my health.

I do not want to be a champion in my 20s, be slower in my 30s and a cripple in my 40s and 50s.

I want it all (greedy I know!).

I want to perform at my peak now PLUS I want to be able

to keep performing into my 30s, 40s, 50s and beyond.

Maybe I will win my age category at Kona or the New York marathon when I am 82 years old—who knows?

My future MUST include:

1. The ability to perform at my peak performance in races now and in the future
2. The ability to maintain (or improve) my fitness with each year
3. As I age, to ensure I maintain my health and avoid (or reduce the risk of) joint replacements, early onset arthritis and diabetes, cancer or heart disease in my 40s and 50s.
4. To reduce or slow down the ageing process

I am sure most of you want the same things too!

There is no point being super fit but looking old and stooped or struggling to get out of a chair at age 48!

Now, of course there is no guarantee. There are many factors at play like genetics, environment, stress and so on. But it is clear that diet does play a significant role in long-term health.

We need to do our part to ensure that the factors that we *do* have control over (i.e. what food we choose to fuel our bodies) help to maintain health and athletic performance and do not contain harmful substances like e-numbers, chemicals and highly processed foods.

What Is The Goal Of This Book?

The goal of this book is to examine the role the ketogenic diet can play in the athlete's diet. It aims to provide some ideas you can use to achieve optimal athletic performance, anti-ageing and better health.

This book will take the research and lessons from scientific studies and apply them to athletic populations to ensure that not only are you able to improve your long-term health but you are also able to gain optimal performance now.

This book aims to share with you stories and anecdotes from current endurance athletes who have embraced the ketogenic lifestyle and have found enormous benefits.

The information in this book is based on the research of PhDs, doctors, scientists and nutritionists from around the world.

I have highlighted many research sources for your reference should you wish to dive deeper into this fascinating subject and start to apply it in your own life.

This is not specific "advice" for you as every individual is different. You will have different a gene profile, different nutritional needs, different family history, allergies and medical issues.

It is up to you to read, get ideas, determine if it resonates with you, do further study and consult with medical professionals (if you have any risk factors) before embarking on any drastic change.

Aims And Objectives

This book aims to bring all the relevant information together in one place. It aims:

1. To examine the ketogenic diet, what it is and how it works
2. To highlight the specific benefits to athletes
3. To outline common mistakes that can be avoided

4. To put together guidelines for optimizing training while on the ketogenic diet

5. To examine the modified ketogenic diet where you can get most of the benefits without being super strict at all times (80/20)

6. To outline what a typical day of eating for an endurance athlete looks like on the ketogenic diet rather than just provide a list of foods

7. To give you all the information you need in one place so you will be able to make an educated decision as to whether this is worth trying for you or not

If you have any questions, please get in touch. I will do my best to help you,

Charlotte
charlotte1@triathlon-hacks.com

Ok, let's get started...

The ketogenic diet is essentially a high-fat, low-carbohydrate, medium-protein diet.

This means instead of eating a high-carb standard American diet (SAD) diet, you switch to eating a very small proportion of carbohydrate, medium amount of protein and high proportion of fat.

Typical proportions of macronutrients in the ketogenic diet are 70-75% fat, 20% protein and 5-10% carbohydrates. These numbers will vary depending on your goals, your current health and your genes.

This is a radical departure from the typical Western diet of 50-60% carbohydrate, 20% protein and 15-20% fat. This turns a lot of traditional beliefs and practices completely on its head.

Since the standard American diet was introduced with its prevalence of refined grains, white potatoes, French fries, and high-sugar drinks, obesity has reached near epidemic proportions and the rates of **type 2 diabetes**, heart disease, stroke and cancer continue to rise.

Polyunsaturated fat and high levels of omega-6 fatty acids compared to omega-3 fatty acids in the Western diet are believed to contribute to autoimmune and inflammatory diseases as well as cancer and cardiovascular disease[81].

We have fallen victim to convenience foods and to marketing and the results are catastrophic!

The Ketogenic Diet Is NOT "New"

The ketogenic diet is not a "new fad diet".

It was designed in 1924 at the Mayo clinic to successfully treat epilepsy. The ketogenic diet radically changes the way that energy is used in the body.

Fat is converted in the liver into fatty acids and ketone bodies. The diet lowers blood glucose levels, improves insulin resistance and teaches the body to prioritize burning fat for fuel instead of glucose.

On the ketogenic diet, a person's body develops the mechanisms to burn and utilize fat more easily for energy through a significant reduction of carbohydrate intake (typically to less than 50 grams per day).

This means the body changes from relying on glycogen as its main source of energy and switches to ketone bodies. In particular, in a keto-adapted (fat-adapted) state, the brain shifts from a sole dependency on glucose to a state where it can also acquire energy from a by-product of fat called beta-hydroxybutyrate.

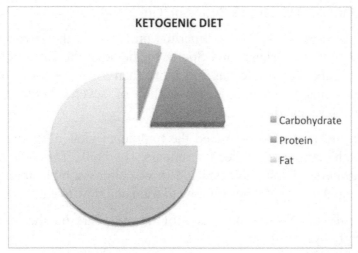

The results can be dramatic. Many studies on the ketogenic diet have demonstrated:

- Dramatic fat loss
- Improved mental clarity
- Reversal of diabetes
- Improved athletic performance

But I'm An Athlete, Not A Lab-Rat! I Need My High Carbohydrate Intake!

Actually, no, it turns out that you don't.

Not so long ago, a low-carbohydrate diet was considered absolutely bonkers for athletes. We "NEEDED" sports drinks, pastas, a 60-70% carbohydrate diet, 6 bowls of cereal for breakfast and pockets full of gels for a long run or ride (or was this just successful marketing)?

It was not just marketing. In fact, very prominent professors and scientists in the running and athletic communities also told us to pump as much carbohydrate into our bodies as possible.

One such person was Professor Tim Noakes.

Professor Noakes is an emeritus professor in the Division of Exercise Science and Sports Medicine at the University of Cape Town. He has run more than 70 marathons and ultra-marathons and is the author of several books on exercise and diet.

In the 1980s, he promoted the traditional view of eating a high carbohydrate diet for runners. His book, *The Lore of Running*[18] (first published 1985), was almost a bible among long distance athletes on how to train and how to eat.

Professor Noakes now says of his 33 years on the high carbohydrate diet:

"I was progressively slower in my running and fatter and ultimately developed type 2 diabetes."

He famously came out recently and said **he was wrong** on his previous views of promoting a high carbohydrate diet. This has resulted in him appearing in court in South Africa to defend his claims against government health officials.

PROFESSOR TIM NOAKES SAYS HE WAS WRONG TO PROMOTE THE HIGH CARBOHYDRATE DIET

Professor Noakes now trains fewer hours and has adopted the ketogenic diet. He has completely reduced his level of injury and burnout.

"The results were dramatic. I lost twenty kilograms of weight...my diabetes is quite well-controlled on Metformin and this low-carbohydrate diet. I realized I had to say sorry that I have been misleading people for so long telling them to eat the high carbohydrate diet."

Further he believes that cutting carbohydrate intake results in no exercise impairment and that the less carbohydrate athletes ingest the better they will perform!

This is a huge departure from traditional wisdom.

Professor Noakes says from his personal experience that he can do any amount of exercise without increasing his carbohydrate intake. He can race up to 21km without needing any more than 50-75 grams of carbohydrate a day in his diet. He does not require supplemental gels or sports drinks.

Professor Noakes now supports the ketogenic way of eating[21] and has a best-selling book, *The Real Meal Revolution*[20], a low-carbohydrate, high-fat (LCHF) diet.

So perhaps we do not need high amounts of carbohydrate to exercise effectively?

6 More Reasons A Ketogenic Diet Will Make You Unstoppable As An Athlete

Rather than the ketogenic diet being "a bit risky" for an athlete to switch to, there seem to be even more reasons to try the ketogenic diet as an athlete!

Better Endurance

Keto-adapted athletes can complete long distances without topping up with extra sugary gels and drinks. This is unthinkable on the traditional athlete's diet.

The traditional athlete's diet says you need to be taking in a sugary gel or sports drink every 30 minutes to stave off "bonking" or running out of energy as the liver only stores enough glycogen for 1-2 hours of exercise.

Even worse for endurance athletes is that it is almost impossible to continually digest more than 200-600 calories as you are exercising. At that rate, you actually cannot physically keep up with your energy demands. This means it is only a matter of time before you run out of energy. If you decide to take on board more fuel than this, the stomach cannot cope and will quickly reject it (read: vomiting at the side of the race).

However, once you become keto-adapted (which means you have trained your body to burn fat for fuel), you no longer require extra glucose top-ups as you have unlimited fuel in the form of body fat. All you tend to need is water and some electrolytes.

Some athletes do actually consume some carbohydrates during ultra-distance racing (>12 hours exercise) but the requirement is significantly less than the traditional athlete's diet.

This significantly reduces the weight you need to carry on long runs or bike rides, which makes you faster. Every gram of weight counts in a race, especially when going uphill.

Plus it also significantly reduces your constant mental calculations about which gel to carry and when to take your next sugar hit.

Reduced Gut Distress

Many triathlon races, ultras or marathons are thwarted by gut pain or diarrhea as you have to gulp down too many sports gels and your stomach protests. Not having to suck down extra calories mid race allows the body to keep the blood flow in the working muscles and not have it partially diverted to the stomach.

This is a massive benefit!

In every Ironman race, 20-30% of the competitors do not finish the event. There are many reasons for this of course, but one of the biggest reasons that great athletes do not complete the event is gut distress. Too many gels and their stomach cannot cope.

Weight Loss

For triathletes, cyclists, runners and most endurance athletes, losing excess body fat results in significantly better performance.

The average Western athlete is generally a bit overweight (even if they are fit) and losing excess body fat immediately results in better performance, faster times, improved health and more energy.

Many athletes, despite their huge amount of exercise, still never lose weight as they are simply burning sugars and replacing sugars with very little nutritional value. Typically, as they train more they get hungrier and eat even more sugars and carbohydrates.

Many athletes never burn any significant amount of fat and, despite their training volume, tend to get fatter each year! One reason for this is that the body prioritizes burning sugar over fat.

Another reason is that when you consume carbohydrates, the body releases insulin in order for glucose to enter cells to be burned for energy. The problem is the action of insulin blocks the breakdown of fat, essentially blocking any fat-burning!

On the ketogenic diet, you eat nutrient dense foods and limit addictive sugars. Most people find they are very rarely, if ever, hungry.

On this diet there is no calorie counting or restriction of calories.

Yay! You eat when you are hungry and do not eat when you are not. Calorie restriction very rarely aids weight loss as the body reacts by slowing the metabolism to conserve fat! Plus calorie restriction sometimes impairs athletic performance and results in loss of muscle mass.

Not a clever strategy!

The focus on the ketogenic diet is a shift in *what* you eat not *how much* you eat.

Increased Energy

Being an athlete involves maintaining a busy schedule trying to fit it all in: job, family, social life and training.

Athletes on the ketogenic diet report less fatigue, more sustainable energy and they find that they can train harder at each session. If each session is more effective, they often find that they can actually train less often, with higher intensity, and reach the same goal. Plus if they have more energy, they get more done and feel better while doing it.

High carbohydrate meals raise the blood sugar levels instantly. This raises insulin levels, stops fat metabolism and promotes fat storage. People experience fatigue and sugar cravings, get distorted hormonal response and finally experience fatigue and burnout.

There must be another way!

Decreased Inflammation

Training creates inflammation in the body. The better athlete you are the more you understand the importance of quick recovery techniques (whether it is ice baths, compression sleeves or sports massages). These all focus on reducing inflammation in the body.

Excess inflammation means you will feel more muscle soreness post exercise, recover slower and feel sluggish.

Excess inflammation also means a higher likelihood of arthritis, cancers, gut disorders, acne and autoimmune diseases in the long-term.

REDUCING INFLAMMATION IS THE KEY TO RECOVERY FOR ATHLETES

It is also the key to good health. Anyone who has researched any diet knows focusing on increasing antioxidants and anti-inflammatory food is the key.

The ketogenic diet is packed with high quality foods, especially vegetables, which contain vitamins, minerals and antioxidants. It focuses on reducing toxic chemicals, preservatives and excessive e-numbers in your foods, which increase inflammation. The ketogenic diet specifically eliminates milk, grains and sugars, which are known to be inflammatory.

Metabolic Flexibility

As I touched on earlier, this is one of the best advantages for athletes. Traditional diets have trained the body to burn sugars for energy. The fat-burning pathway has largely been forgotten. As you exercise and run out of glycogen/sugar, you must keep topping up with more sugar to prevent running out of fuel.

If you are a sugar burner, your body simply cannot access the huge amounts of energy contained in your body fat. Fat is an almost unlimited source of energy, yielding 4000 calories for every pound (lb.) of fat.

Metabolic flexibility means that the body can easily burn whichever fuel source is available. Instead of having to top up every half hour with another gel, the body simply burns the fat it is already carrying, which is readily available.

As you train on the ketogenic diet you get better and better at burning fat for energy instead of sugars. When you can access your fat-burning pathways, you can virtually keep going forever without refuelling.

Even the skinniest single digit body fat athlete carries enough fat to produce 40,000 calories. (This means most of us have substantially more!)

Professor Tim Noakes explains[21], "By keeping carbs below 25g a day, the body moves from a carb burning state to a fat-burning state. Ketones are formed when fatty acids are broken down by the liver for energy.

"These molecules are generated during fat metabolism –
and are a sign that your body is now using fat for energy.
This process forces the body to burn fat."

Therapeutic Uses Of The Ketogenic Diet

There is dramatic research in the therapeutic uses of the
ketogenic diet such as reversing and improving diabetes[22],
cancers[23, 24, 25], epilepsy[26] and other chronic diseases on the
ketogenic diet. Many diabetics can completely get off
medication or significantly reduce it.

If you can still exercise at the same or better level of
performance and avoid the significant action of
"carbohydrate which contributes to progressive weight
gain, continual hunger, lethargy and, in time, pancreatic
failure and the onset of adult-onset diabetes"[19], why
wouldn't you?

More research needs to be done into cancer prevention and
treatment, but there are strong indications the ketogenic
diet may play an important role.

This book will not explore therapeutic uses of the ketogenic
diet, as that is a whole book in itself, but it will make you
aware of the added benefits. You can do more research into
this if one of these areas is relevant to you.

The aim of the ketogenic diet is to get into nutritional ketosis. This is a state where the liver breaks down fat into ketones, which are then burned for energy.

(Please note that this is NOT keto-acidosis, which is a dangerous condition for type 1 diabetics. It is a sign of insufficient insulin and is associated with rapid breathing, flushed cheeks, abdominal pain, acetone on the breath (bad breath), dehydration and vomiting.)

What Is Nutritional Ketosis?

Nutritional ketosis is a state of health in which your body is efficiently burning fat as its primary fuel source instead of glucose. The term "nutritional ketosis" is claimed to have been coined by Dr. Stephen Phinney & Dr. Jeff Volek, two of the leading experts[1] and researchers in the field of low carbohydrate dieting.

BY BURNING FAT INSTEAD OF SUGARS, YOU TAP INTO AN ALMOST UNLIMITED SOURCE OF SUSTAINABLE ENERGY THROUGHOUT THE DAY

You will lose the sugar highs and lows and just feel consistently great with enough energy to train, to work, to have family time and perform better.

You will notice that you lose that "foggy-brain" feeling mid-afternoon when most people experience a sugar low and can barely drag themselves through the afternoon.

When you achieve nutritional ketosis by following the ketogenic diet, you are essentially converting yourself from a "sugar burner" to a "fat burner".

This is accomplished by reducing your consumption of carbohydrates, increasing your intake of fat, and consuming only an adequate amount of protein to meet your body's needs.

Over a span of a few weeks, the body "up-regulates" the enzymes and other "metabolic machinery" needed to burn fat more efficiently, therefore making it easier for your body to tap into stored fat as an energy source.

How Do You Know If You're In Nutritional Ketosis?

Ketosis is actually a natural state to be in.

WE ARE ALL IN KETOSIS FIRST THING IN THE MORNING AS WE HAVE FASTED OVERNIGHT

If you had dinner by 7:30pm and did not eat again until 7:30am the next morning, you underwent a 12-hour fast and were in nutritional ketosis until you ate breakfast.

Ketosis is not an artificial state. You can live for 40-60 days with no food precisely because you can turn fat into ketones for fuel. If you had to rely purely on glucose, you would be dead in a few days.

If you had to rely purely on protein, you would be dead in a few more days but have wasted muscles. Here is a fascinating study where a man did a medically supervised fast for 382 days[38] with no ill-effects. He had just water and electrolytes.

Human beings survived for millennia by being in ketosis. In the days when food was scare and the next meal was uncertain, nutritional ketosis allowed people to survive for days or weeks on very little, if any, food.

They could do this by the body switching to its natural energy source of stored fat. Most of these ancient people were not fat! Yet even the leanest people have enough stored body fat to provide sufficient energy to survive for weeks.

When you are in ketosis, your body is running on ketone bodies as fuel. By measuring your ketone levels, you will be able to confirm whether you are in ketosis.

There are 3 types of ketone bodies:

- Acetoacetate (AcAc)
- Beta-hydroxybutyrate (BHB) and
- Acetone

In your blood, you can measure all 3 ketone bodies. In your urine, AcAc and acetone can be measured. And in your breath you can measure acetone.

Your blood ketone levels are the best indicator of ketosis. Unfortunately, measuring blood ketone levels is also the most expensive method and least practical.

Most people measure their urine and breath ketone levels instead. Ketostix are a well-known brand in this space. You will need to test more frequently in the beginning (once or twice a day) as you adapt to the ketogenic diet.

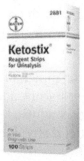

When you are first starting a low-carb or ketogenic diet and are transitioning into ketosis from a moderate to high-carb diet, Ketostix strips will confirm that your body has in fact done what biology says that it must do. It will show that your liver has begun producing ketones.

Once you're in ketosis and are becoming fat-adapted, you won't need to test as often. In fact, it becomes unreliable to test once you are fat-adapted as Ketostix only measures *excess* levels of acetoacetate.

This tends not to be excreted as you adapt as the muscles convert it to beta-hydroxybutyrate and return it to the blood for use by the brain.

Ketostix will measure excess ketones that are in your urine. However, they are not the be all and end all of being in ketosis. You can be in ketosis and not have ketones in your urine if you are using all your ketones for energy or if you're getting rid of the excess through sweat or saliva. The ketostix reading may be negative. Keep this in mind and do not obsess about them. Use them as a guide.

As you understand the diet better and stabilize your ketone levels you will be able to feel more quickly (without testing) when you have dropped out of ketosis.

If you consume too many carbohydrates, you will be kicked out of ketosis temporarily. However, if you once again restrict carbohydrates, you will go right back into ketosis within 24 hours.

This is because the liver can store only a small amount of glycogen. When you restrict carbohydrates, the liver will run out of glycogen within a day and begin burning fat instead (which is turned into ketones).

If you have a medical condition that makes monitoring

blood ketone levels necessary or if you are a numbers geek with a bit of spending money, you may be interested in purchasing a ketone blood meter and test strips for measuring beta hydroxybutyrate in your blood. The test strips cost somewhere between $2 and $5 per strip.

Nutritional ketosis is achieved when your blood ketones are between 0.5 and 3.0 mol/L. Values higher than that have no additional benefits. Over 0.5 mmol/L on the meter is entry level nutritional ketosis but 1.5 – 3 mmol/L is considered 'optimal ketosis'.

There are a few meters to choose from:

Precision Xtra[27]

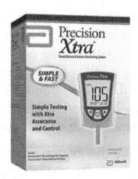

Nova Max Plus[28]

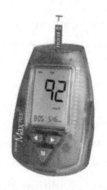

Is Being In Ketosis A Binary "All Or Nothing" State?

Being on a low-carbohydrate diet has fantastic health benefits and is a sliding scale. It is not an "all-or-nothing" state.

You can be on a low-carb diet to varying degrees.

But being in nutritional ketosis is a binary state.
Either you are or you aren't.
(Just like being pregnant!)

Dr. Peter Attia, an expert in the ketogenic diet has this advice[29]:

"For most people, a gradual reduction in carbs, beginning with the worst offenders (sugar and highly refined and processed grains) yields fantastic results, including fat loss, reduction in triglycerides, increase in size and maturity of HDL and reduction of LDL particles number."

DR. ATTIA SAYS IF YOUR DIET IS FULL OF SUGARS, YOU ARE NOT DOING YOURSELF ANY FAVORS, NO MATTER WHAT DIET YOU ARE ON

So even if you feel the strict ketogenic diet is too much for you, he suggests you still make an effort to reduce sugar (carbohydrate) consumption to gain some of the dramatic health benefits.

Sugar gets metabolized at the expense of everything else. So whatever you eat with sugar is unlikely to get metabolized. In the late 1960s, John Yudkin[30] published a study suggesting that it was pretty harmful to eat "lots" of sugar with fat (maybe even worse than just sugar alone, and certainly worse than fat alone, which causes no harm).

You can also watch this lecture[31] Dr. Lustig gave in 2009 called **Sugar: The Bitter Truth** (watched nearly 7 million times).

Dr. Attia advises that you keep your diet simple. If you are avoiding sugars and highly refined carbs, the only thing else you need to think about (fat-wise) is reducing your intake of omega-6 fatty acids.

If I Am In Nutritional Ketosis Does This Mean That I Am Now Fat-Adapted?

There is a difference between being in ketosis and being fat-adapted. Being in ketosis means you have ketones in circulation. To know for sure, you will need to measure with the methods I discussed above.

If you think you have been in ketosis for 2 weeks but are not losing weight or feeling better, it is likely that you are not in ketosis quite yet. Measure your ketone levels to get objective results.

Being keto-adapted or fat-adapted means your body has built the metabolic machinery and is primed to digest and metabolize fat as its primary energy source with very little glucose.

If you limit carbohydrates, you will be in ketosis in less than 24 hours but the changes of keto-adaptation occur at the DNA level and involve changes in enzyme expression and mitochondrial function. These may take up to 8-12 weeks to occur.

Many people on the standard American diet (SAD) wake up in ketosis every day purely through not eating overnight. But this does not mean they are fat-adapted. To achieve this requires being in ketosis for an extended period of time to provide the stimulus for your body to alter its metabolic expression profile.

Ketosis means that your body is breaking down fat at such a rate that there are ketones in your bloodstream. This happens after fasting or over time with a low carbohydrate diet.

KETOSIS IS A NORMAL METABOLIC STATE

If you've ever had steak and veggies for supper and then had eggs for breakfast (or skipped it all together) you've been in ketosis.

It's also important to note that your body burns whatever fuel is available—glucose, FFA (free fatty acids), ketones or alcohol. Your body will burn sugars first even if there is available fat.

When you first enter ketosis, you are using fat for energy, but at first it's in limited amounts because you don't have as many fat-converting enzymes. These get built up over time. This is what causes the tiredness at the beginning of the diet.

Once the enzymes are in place, your cells change the way they get energy. It's really amazing to consider all the changes that have to happen internally for keto-adaptation to happen.

Once you are keto-adapted (which can take a few weeks to a few months depending on the person), fat/ketones becomes the preferred fuel. Hormone levels change, glycogen is lowered, and you will carry less excess water. You're able to function well with lots of energy. You can exercise, lift, build up endurance and will have improved mental clarity.

When you're keto-adapted and get an "overdose" of carbs (more than your body needs at the time) different things happen. First, glycogen gets replenished, which causes water retention. Secondly, insulin rises, which can affect other hormone levels as well. While your body processes the carbs, you are not burning ketones.

Once the glucose is dealt with, you will go back into ketosis. When you're keto-adapted, this doesn't take long because you already have the enzymes and are "primed" to use fat for energy.

When you're starting a ketogenic diet for the first time, you do not have these fat-burning enzymes built up already as you have been a sugar burner.

The more often you "fall off the wagon" in the beginning and have sugar the longer it takes to become keto-adapted. When you are keto-adapted, sugar will still take precedence over fat for fuel (because excess blood sugar is fatal and so your body *needs* to handle the sugar first).

Grains and Sugars: The Major Culprits

The most powerful thing about the ketogenic diet is massively reducing sugar (carbohydrates).

Sugar and processed carbohydrates actually change the biochemistry in our bodies so that we crave more, eat more, gain fat and develop insulin resistance and potentially diabetes BECAUSE of our over-exposure to sugar.

The worst part is that sugar is everywhere in processed foods, from ketchup to juice to pasta sauce to bread to cold cut meats.

This is so much more effective for weight loss than those diets that say you can eat anything you want as long as you don't go over 1500 calories. These diets tend not to work long term.

"Low-fat diets are counterproductive," says Eleftheria Maratos-Flier[32], director of obesity research at Harvard's prestigious Joslin Diabetes Center. "They have the paradoxical effect of making people gain weight."

Traditional Diet

As an example, a typical breakfast of juice, bagel, cereal and skim milk is essentially *four cups full of sugar* and sugar-like highly processed carbohydrates.

And for athletes, that's *before* you consume the sugary gels and sports drinks that so many endurance athletes consume every day.

What a way to welcome diabetes and obesity early into your life!

Dependence on sugar is linked to a wide variety of disorders, from symptoms such as poor energy, intestinal bloating, hormone imbalance and increased body fat to diseases such as type 2 diabetes, Alzheimer's and heart disease.

Dr. Peter Attia, also a great endurance athlete, says about pasta, rice and corn, "I view those foods the way I view cigarettes. Literally. I'm totally starch-free. And obviously I consume no sugar."

On this traditionally carbohydrate-rich diet, this is what happens when you exercise:

Dietary carbohydrates (grains, fruit, starchy veggies, juice and sport drinks) are processed then stored in the liver and muscles as glycogen. During exercise, these glycogen stores fuel our working muscles.

The harder the workout the quicker these glycogen stores get depleted. Glycogen stores are limited, so during exercise lasting more than 60-90 minutes, you have to continue consuming carbohydrates while exercising to maintain the fuel source or you experience "bonking", i.e. running out of energy where you literally cannot continue until you ingest more sugar.

More specifically, 30-60g of carbohydrate per hour is required to keep you fuelled and feeling strong. So a typical athlete might ingest 2 Clif bars and 3 gels during a 90-minute ride.

Sound familiar?

Hence the reliance on external carbohydrates during long bouts of exercise and the proliferation of advice to take one gel every 30 minutes in an Ironman and to continue drinking carbohydrate throughout.

One of the biggest problems in a long-distance race is stomach upsets and GI distress due to too many gels and sugary drinks.

Burning glycogen has other problems too. It is toxic in excess and it's an inflammatory substance. It is a cheap source of fuel but it is not clean and offers minimal nutrition.

There is no good reason to consume excessive carbohydrates.

Grains, in particular, irritate the gut and create excessive inflammation within the body. When many people stop eating grains, it is common to hear that many of their symptoms like leaky gut syndrome, IBS and other intestinal disorders miraculously disappear.

Is It Possible To Correct Leaky Gut Syndrome?

A lot of athletes put a ton of rubbish food in their body, often too many grains, sugars and chemicals. Even if you are not gluten intolerant, it is still possible to get inflammatory changes or gut irritation from too many grains.

Maybe you do not suffer gut distress on a normal day but suffer on race day from an overload of having to put more fuel in your stomach than it can handle.

If, instead, you teach your body to access the fat it is already carrying, you reduce this distress instantly.

It does not mean you can never take supplementary fuel. Used wisely, carbohydrates will give you a boost for sure.

BUT IF YOU CAN TRAIN YOURSELF NOT TO *RELY* ON THEM AND JUST USE THEM STRATEGICALLY, YOU WILL EFFECTIVELY HAVE A SECRET WEAPON AT YOUR DISPOSAL

It depends how fat-adapted you are and the length of your race.

Some 100-mile ultra-athletes do allow themselves a couple of gels at mile 60 or 70, but this is vastly different to requiring one every half hour.

If you are not yet fully fat-adapted, you might be able to reduce your intake of supplementary gels to 40-50% of what you used to require until you gradually are able to reduce it more. This will require testing during training as you progress with your diet.

Any reduction in your body's demands for extra food intake will help you in training and racing. It is difficult for the body to divert blood and energy to the stomach to process fuel when all the blood is out supplying the working muscles.

Studies have looked at endurance runners and found that the majority have blood in their stool at the end of a long training run or a long race[33].

There is no doubt that there is gut distress during a long event. By being able to access your fat stores, you may not eliminate this completely but you can massively reduce it.

Biochemistry On The Ketogenic Diet And Why It Makes Sense

The ketogenic diet provides incredible metabolic flexibility. This means the body can burn either fat or sugar, whatever is available.

If there is no sugar available in the bloodstream, the body will use fat to burn as a source of energy.

Fat is a cleaner energy source and a more efficient energy source than sugar. It produces more energy per gram. 1 gram of fat has 9 calories, while carbohydrates produce just 4 calories per gram.

BURNING FAT IS BY FAR THE MOST EFFICIENT ENERGY TO BURN

We all have a lot of fat on hand as available fuel. Even the leanest triathlete or marathon runner has enough fat to fuel multiple Ironman races or ultras back to back without running out of fuel.

Imagine if we could easily access that

If you are currently a sugar burner, your body will not be used to accessing the fat stores and pretty quickly it will just run out of glucose and stop.

But with the ketogenic diet and correct training, the body is able to rebuild the metabolic machinery to process and access these fat stores to give you a virtually unlimited energy supply.

Dr. Phinney and Dr. Volek have been studying [1,2] the low carbohydrate diet with athletes since the 1980s. They produced great results early on but most of the studies only lasted 6-7 days as the athletes were so obsessed with eating carbohydrates that it was difficult to find subjects who were willing to try it for extended periods of time.The results were interesting at the time but not significant.

Now, however, the results are undeniable. Drs. Phinney and Volek have now tested athletes who have been eating low carbohydrate diets for 2 years and more. They are seeing doubling of fat utilisation levels at VO2 max. They are reporting significant increases in power generated[34].

So whilst in the past it was thought that the body prefers to burn glycogen, actually fat is the preferred source, if it is allowed to be.

The ketogenic diet offers an exciting new frontier in athletic performance and disease prevention. Ketogenic and low carbohydrate athletes are performing amazing feats of endurance by remaining in a fat-burning state.

As Dr. Lili-Williams[35] summarizes, from current research studies, the metabolic benefits to endurance athletes may include increased ATP and mitochondria production, efficient fatty acid oxidation, and maybe VO2 max increase.

How long will it take to see results?

The primary goal of a ketogenic diet and aerobic training is to build up your metabolic machinery to easily access and burn fat for energy. This will take several weeks to several months as you have likely been a sugar burner for many years.

You still have to do the work and train the body (more on this later) to adapt to burning fat. You cannot just drink exogenous ketones or take a tablet and get the result in a day. So, like anything sustainable, there is no quick fix or tablet to take. ☺

Within 4-8 weeks, you should notice 80% of benefits, though it may take a few months to fully adapt.

Specific Adaptations For Athletes

As with any diet, you need to implement the basics then test it and tweak it:

- For your body
- For your sport

Athletes have different requirements to the standard sedentary population.

The advice for most people who want results on a ketogenic diet is to consume no more than 25-50g of carbohydrate a day. This is a good figure to aim for in the beginning to get into nutritional ketosis.

Later on, depending on your training, you might be able to eat 100-150g of carbohydrate a day and still be in ketosis.

In general, men can eat more carbohydrate than women and still be in ketosis due to a higher muscle mass.

As a general rule, Mark Sisson, in his book *Primal*

Endurance[36] (2016), suggests athletes should aim to eat:

- Less than 100g carbohydrate a day if you are aiming to lose fat
- Around 150g carbohydrate a day for maintenance
- If you go above 150g you may experience gradual weight gain
- If you go above 300g carbohydrate a day you will be moving towards chronic disease

Depending on your physiology, you might be able to have 40g of carbohydrate daily and remain in ketosis. Some people can have 130g of carbohydrate and remain in ketosis. The average person on the standard Western diet consumes 300-450g a day.

As always in the beginning, track your food, your performance, how you feel, how you sleep and how you perform. Allow 4-6 weeks to adapt before giving up!

Many athletes allow themselves to have 50-100g of carbohydrate before and after particularly hard training sessions but limit carbohydrates the rest of the week.

There is increasing evidence that the ketogenic diet is perfect for endurance athletes.

But What About Sprint Athletes Or Power Lifting Athletes?

Menno Henselman has written extensively[5] about this. He is a bodybuilder who does a cyclic ketogenic diet. He goes in and out of ketosis depending on his competition cycles. Even building muscle while in ketosis is possible.

He believes both strength training and endurance training are perfectly suited to a ketogenic diet.

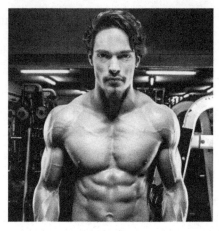

Here are some of his guidelines for the cyclic ketogenic diet. Many strength training athletes and body builders are reporting fantastic results from the ketogenic diet. Also strength training is vitally important to endurance athletes as well. If you are an endurance athlete but not doing strength training, you need to start!

Cyclic Ketogenic Diet

The standard format for a cyclical ketogenic diet is 5-6 days of ketogenic dieting and 1-2 days of high carbohydrate eating. It has been followed extensively by the strength training community for many years for effective fat loss and simultaneous muscle gain. This "re-feed" is good for hormonal balance and thyroid activity. Dr. Phinney and Dr. Volek also agree that cycling in and out of ketosis is the best way to sustain the benefits of the ketogenic diet over the long term.

The cyclical ketogenic diet is generally easier to maintain as it devotes one to two **FULL** days of high carbohydrate consumption in order to fully refill muscle glycogen stores. This means that the cyclic ketogenic diet is not for beginners that are unable to perform the necessary amount or intensity of training. You must **completely** deplete glycogen stores each week in order to have a successful cyclic ketogenic diet.

Rather than go into the complexities of each of these diets, most people only require a standard ketogenic diet. Most people reading this will not yet be advanced in the ketogenic diet.

Unless you have already successfully done a ketogenic diet for 2 years or more and understand it, do not over complicate it.

Menno's advice: During hard core weight training, if you do not feel like you will die during your workout, you do not need extra carbs. If you do feel like you will collapse and die, you may have 20g before your workout.

According to Menno, the ketogenic diet is great for sprinters, body builders and endurance athletes. However, it may not work as well for 400-800m runners due to different energy requirements.

Back To The Endurance World

Back to the endurance world, Zach Bitter[37], holder of the 12-hour world record and 100-mile American record (and many other titles) has an interesting take on the ketogenic diet.

He does not stress about the strict definition. His diet is high fat, low carbohydrate but he feels the exact amounts differ widely for each individual.

His goal is not "to be in ketosis" but to perform better (like most of us ultimately!).

Phinney and Volek[1, 2] state that to be ketogenic you must be under 50g carbohydrate. Zach, however, is often over that but admittedly he does far more exercise than the standard person and is super active.

He uses nutritional ketosis as his guiding principle but is not a slave to it. In fact, he uses carbohydrates like a stimulant. When used properly, they can give you a much-needed boost. When abused, they leave you "wrecked, burnt out and puking up gels."

This sounds like a sensible approach.

What About "Carbing Up" Prior To An Endurance Event?

If you are doing a 1-2 hour event, this is completely unnecessary. However, if you are running 100 miles or any hard endurance work over 3 hours, a "carb boost" during the event may help you.

There is no "need" for a carbo-loading, even with endurance sports, but some people find the boost helpful depending on their goals and how fat-adapted they are.

Dr. Peter Attia doesn't use any extra carbs unless he is cycling hard for more than 3 hours. If so, he will allow himself some carbs as a boost when needed.

So, if you are exercising for less than 3 hours, aim not to ingest any extra carbs.

What is certain is that you do not need carb top-ups every half hour!

Can A Vegetarian Do The Ketogenic Diet?

Yes, vegetarians can do the ketogenic diet. Being in ketosis requires a lot of fat. It is relatively easy to find fat in animal products, but here are some good non-meat sources:

It depends if you include dairy and eggs in your vegetarian diet. For those that do, the following are helpful:

1. Eggs and egg yolks provide a significant amount of healthy fat and are very nutrient-dense with basically no carbohydrates present.

2. Raw (unpasteurized) cheese made from the milk of cows that are pastured (they only roam the pasture eating grass) and fed 100% grass provides significant amounts of fat with little to no carbohydrates, along with a plethora of other nutrients as well as bacteria for the bowels.

3. Heavy cream is a welcome addition to many cups of morning coffee because it provides a hefty amount of fat with little to no protein or carbohydrates, as well as conjugated linoleic acid (if from cows that eat grass and not grains or corn).

What About A Vegan?

Getting fat from non-animal sources[40]:

Eat plenty of good oils, vegetables, some fruits, and nuts:

1. Avocados, which are actually a fruit, provide a healthy amount of monounsaturated fat, a plethora of vitamins and nutrients, and most of the carbohydrate content is fiber, which feeds your bowel bacteria and will not affect ketone levels like non-fiber carbohydrates.

2. Coconuts, coconut oil, and coconut manna (the pulp of the coconut which contains some fiber) provide significant saturated fat and medium-chain triglycerides, which are easily turned into ketones.

3. Macadamia nuts provide the best bang for your buck in terms of fat-to-carbohydrate ratios with 21 grams of fat per ounce serving and only four grams of carbs (two

grams are fiber).

4. Almonds are also good sources of fat and vitamins but can often lead to issues, as their fat content per ounce serving drops to 14 grams and the carbohydrates rise to six grams.

Add oils to your cooking to increase the fat content. Good suggestions include: Coconut oil, olive oil (make sure it is fresh as it spoils quickly and avoid high heat), macadamia oil, ghee or butter (100% grass-fed and raw if possible).

How Does A Vegetarian Get Enough Protein On The Ketogenic Diet?

Unless you eat eggs and/or dairy, it's difficult to meet your daily protein requirements on a vegetarian keto diet plan. Do not underestimate the importance of sufficient protein. It's as important as your carb intake. Insufficient protein will result in muscle loss. You will burn fewer calories at rest and feel hungrier.

Although fat makes a low-carb diet filling, studies show that protein is the most sating macronutrient by far. A common mistake for low-carbers is that they eat less protein in fear that they will go out of ketosis (as a result of gluconeogenesis).

However, the truth is that you'd have to eat significantly more protein consistently to disrupt ketosis. Finally, your daily protein requirements will vary based on your activity and lifestyle.

Make sure you know your ideal "average" protein intake.

Vegetables generally contain more carbohydrates than meat sources, especially the fatty cuts of meat that are generally consumed on a ketogenic diet. As vegetarians must rely on increased amounts of vegetables and fruits, extra care must be taken to keep the carbohydrates limited.

Leafy greens and cruciferous vegetables are great sources of nutrients, and they can be cooked or garnished in fatty sources or eaten in a salad with olive oil. This will increase the amount of fat in the diet.

Fruits should be watched closely and the best sources seem to be berries as the skin is consumed and made mostly of fiber. These include blueberries, strawberries, raspberries, and blackberries. Fruits like bananas are difficult to eat on a full ketogenic diet as they can contain large amounts of carbohydrates and sugar and are therefore best avoided.

Whether you are a carnivore or vegetarian, ketosis is a normal state that your body encounters. If you are planning on undergoing a full-blown ketogenic diet or periodic ketosis, you are able to do it without meat as part of your diet.

As always, track your macro (fat, carbohydrate or protein) intake and measure results.

Intermittent fasting (IF) is one of those topics that are gaining quickly in popularity.

There is a ton of research into it and the benefits are phenomenal.

The main factor that stops many people considering fasting is the fear and discomfort of being hungry.

For athletes in particular, it is the fear of poor performance — not having enough energy on board and "bonking", being unable to finish your race or training session.

For strength training athletes, it is the fear of losing muscle mass.

HOWEVER, THE BEAUTY OF INTERMITTENT FASTING IS YOU GAIN ALL THE BENEFITS WITHOUT EXTREME HUNGER OR A DIP IN PERFORMANCE

It does not mean going on a week-long fast.

One protocol many people have that is fairly easy is a 16-hour daily fast. You consume all your calories in an 8-hour period. Basically, you easily achieve this if you skip breakfast. You stop eating by 8pm at night then skip breakfast and do not eat again until lunchtime at around 12pm[41].

For 10-12 hours of this fasting period you are (hopefully) asleep.
If this is too hard initially, do it gradually.
First reduce snacking between meals.
Then keep delaying breakfast by 1 hour a day until you are

on the "16-hour fast" schedule.

Benefits of Intermittent Fasting:

Save Time

Even simple meals have setup time, eating time and clear up time. Completely eliminating one meal will save you at least an hour a day.

Skipping breakfast will also eliminate decision-making expenditure. Even if is simple, there is still decision making to be done at breakfast time:

- What do I feel like eating?
- What should I be eating?
- What have I got on today?
- How hungry am I?

Instead, get up and get on with your day and do not think about food until lunchtime.

Live Longer

It is scientifically undisputed[42] that restricting calories helps you live longer. Intermittent fasting activates the same mechanisms for extending life as calorie restriction. This is great as it enables you to get the amazing health benefits without the misery of hunger and calorie restriction.

Beneficial changes occur in several genes and molecules related to longevity and protection against disease.

Prevent Cancer

There is growing evidence that intermittent fasting may kill off/clean up pre-cancerous cells that we all have floating around after the age of 40yrs, if not before.

Fasting triggers a metabolic pathway called autophagy, which removes waste material from cells[43].

Intermittent fasting has also been shown to reduce the nasty side effects of chemotherapy.

Lower Your Risk Of Diabetes

Studies on intermittent fasting show 3-6% decrease in fasting blood sugar levels and 20-31% decrease in fasting insulin levels[44]. Blood levels of insulin drop significantly, which facilitates fat burning.

Get Lean

This is not through calorie restriction but your body initiates important cellular repair processes and changes hormone levels to make stored body fat more accessible.

Intermittent fasting puts your body in a fat-burning state. Blood insulin levels drop[45] and growth hormone production increases[46] contributing to fat loss and muscle gain.

Easy To Stick To

Intermittent fasting is much easier to do long term than traditional diets as you are not in starvation mode, nor are you calorie restricting.

In fact, you should get into ketosis much more quickly and then feel an abundance of energy.

Reduce Oxidative Stress And Inflammation

Oxidative stress and inflammation are significantly involved in the ageing process, chronic disease and poor recovery from exercise[47].

Intermittent fasting may induce important cellular repair processes, such as removing waste material from cells. There are also beneficial changes in several genes and molecules related to longevity and protection against disease

Autophagy Switched On

Autophagy is important in the process of preventing cancer. It is a normal process where cells recycle waste material and repair themselves. This is required to maintain muscle mass, slow the ageing process and aid mental health.

And best of all, intermittent fasting stimulates these processes without requiring a 3-day fast.

Intermittent Fasting Timing-How Long And How Often?

Intermittent fasting can be used once you are fat-adapted to accelerate fat loss, slow the ageing process, assist the insulin response, improve cellular repair and boost immunity.

In fact, make a conscious effort not to eat any meal throughout the day until you are actually hungry.

It is quite easy to move to just 2 meals a day.

If this is working for you, you can try to move to 1 meal a day later on.

Do these things slowly, do not change too quickly or your body will resist. You will not be able to sustain it.

The problem for most of the Western world is too much food, not lack of food. We eat due to boredom; we eat because of sugar addiction; we eat because a clock has reached a certain number whether we are hungry or not.

Aim to become more mindful of chewing your food properly and enjoying it, not just gulping it down mindlessly.

If you think about it, intermittent fasting was the way we evolved to eat. This was no doubt the way we existed for millions of years when we had to forage for food. Humans could only eat when they caught something or collected it.

No doubt there were plenty of times when they went without a meal and their bodies were built to cope with this. Modern convenience foods are only a very recent phenomenon that has been accompanied by an astronomic rise in diabetes, heart disease, cancer and stroke.

Food exists to provide us energy, not to relieve boredom.

EVEN THE SKINNIEST TRIATHLETE HAS ENOUGH BODY FAT TO LAST THROUGH FIVE BACK-TO-BACK ULTRA MARATHONS

We can certainly skip a meal now and then and be absolutely fine.

Intermittent fasting will speed up your journey to becoming keto-adapted. But make sure you are getting all your macros. Do not calorie restrict overall.

I don't recommend that you go straight for a 1-2 day fast, but begin by restricting yourself to certain eating windows.

We discussed the 16-hour fast/8 hour eating. This is actually quite easy.

When you have tried this for a few weeks and are used to it, you can experiment with the fasting window.

Other popular protocols athletes follow are the 21/3, which is 21 hours fasting, 3 hours feeding, or the 19/5: 19 hours fasting and 5 hours feeding.

Some people do a 24-hour fast once a week or once a month. Most athletes do not do this one as it can interrupt training. If you wish to try this (it has great health benefits) it is best to have your rest day on a fasting day or do it in the off-season.

On any fasting regimen, continue to monitor your weight and body fat percentage. If you are already very lean, you may not wish to lose much more. Be clear what your goals are and monitor accordingly.

Your body will adjust itself to fasting, and you will find yourself not as hungry as you used to be (especially when you lose the sugar cravings). Make sure you properly record and maintain your total nutrient levels.

In this fasting state, your body can break down extra fat that's stored for the energy it needs. When you're in ketosis, your body already mimics a fasting state, being that you already have little to no glucose in your bloodstream, so you use the fat in your body as energy.

Intermittent fasting uses the same reasoning—instead of using the fats you are eating to gain energy you are using your stored fat. So intermittent fasting can accelerate the benefits gained form ketosis.

Intermittent Fasting For Endurance Athletes

Any diet must be easy to do and be simple. If you have to think too much about it, you will not keep it up. Also, if you are already very lean or if you are doing ultra-endurance events, if may not be right for you.

Zach Bitter describes his experience[48] where his training mileage is so great fasting would hinder instead of aid his progress.

He is an ultra runner and feels that with such a long regular fast it becomes almost impossible for him to get enough calories in.

So it will be different for everyone. Experiment and see what works for you. If you have excess weight to lose, it may be a great way to shed extra fat quickly.

It seems like there are more health benefits to be had rather than performance gains benefits. However, for me, I am determined to do everything possible to prevent cancers, stroke, diabetes and other modern illnesses; I believe intermittent fasting is an easy way to allow the body to have a break and clean up some toxins, dead cells and activate good hormones.

It is also the quickest way to stimulate fat-burning mechanisms, which will enhance performance.

Dr. John Berardi, Chief Science Officer of Precision Nutrition[49], has followed the growing popularity of intermittent fasting as it rises to mythical heights. He decided to test it. Over 6 months, he dropped 20 pounds from 190lbs to 170lbs and went from 10% body fat to 4% body fat whilst maintain lean body mass.

Overall he says it is not for everyone. It is interesting and may help you in the short term. It is not completely necessary to be healthy. Other diet protocols may suit you better. He made an interesting point that fasting teaches you the difference between body hunger and mental hunger.

This in itself, even done short term, is a useful exercise!

Greg McMillan[68] from Mcmillian running is also a big believer in reducing reliance on sugar for energy. He also suggests a program of not eating before a long slow run so that there are very few carbohydrates on hand and your body is encouraged to access its own fat stores for energy.

He suggests not topping up with sugary gels or drinks during these runs. Take water with electrolytes so you do not get dehydrated.

It takes practice for your body to adapt. So do not make a sudden change if you have never done this before. Get up and do a slow run before you eat in the morning and gradually extend your distance without carbohydrates. Take some gels with you just in case you are over optimistic or are out longer than expected.

Ok, sounds good but what are the specifics—how do I start?

In this chapter, I will address specifics and outline a step-by-step plan to help you get started.

Obviously you will need to adapt it to your stage of training and any particular dietary requirements you have.

Specific Foods You Can And Can't Eat On The Ketogenic Diet

Firstly, here is a list of the "allowed" foods:

You Can Eat:

All vegetables (except potato, sweet potato and parsnips as these are high in carbohydrates): Leafy, green vegetables are excellent like cabbage, lettuce, spinach, kale.

Other vegetables: artichoke hearts, asparagus, aubergines, avocados, broccoli, Brussels sprouts, cauliflower, celery courgettes, leeks, mushrooms, olives, onions, peppers, pumpkin, radishes sauerkraut, spring onions, tomatoes

All meats including beef, fish, chicken, pork, shellfish, lobster, squid. Organ meats (brain, heart, liver, kidney, tripe) are the most nutritious meat on offer and worth considering. If you cook them up in a dish with herbs and spices and some vegetables, they actually taste ok!

Do not eat swordfish and tilefish due to their high mercury content. All natural and cured meats are allowed (pancetta, Parma ham, coppa etc.) All natural and cured sausages are allowed (salami, chorizo).

Oily fish like sardines and mackerel are a ketogenic super food. They involve no preparation and can be eaten straight from the tin as a nutritious snack or prepared as a nutritious meal. They are packed with many good fats.

Fats: These must make up the majority of your diet. Avocado oil, ghee, coconut oil, olive oil, macadamia oil, duck fat, butter, sesame oil (small amounts only), MCT (medium chain triglyceride) oil.

So even though the ketogenic diet is all about eating a high proportion of fat in your diet, the type of fat is very important.

This diet does not allow gorging on McDonald's and KFC! Get your fats from oily fish, good oils, meat and eggs, avocados.

Snacks: Nuts and seeds in moderation. Macadamia nuts, pecan nuts, pine nuts, pumpkin seeds, sunflower seeds, and walnuts are all very nutritious. Do not overeat nuts as some of them contain a high proportion of carbohydrates. Flaxseeds are good too but watch out for pre-ground flaxseeds, they go rancid quickly and become toxic.

Other good snacks include small amount of dark chocolate, beef jerky, and any egg dishes.

Drinks: Coconut milk, almond milk, cashew milk, broth (or bouillon) coffee (no sugar!), tea, herbal teas, water, lemon and lime juice (small amounts), club soda, sparkling mineral water.

Dairy: Be careful with dairy. Many people are lactose intolerant and do not know it. It is best to eliminate it for a month and see how you feel. Later, you can slowly introduce it and track your energy and performance levels.

If you do choose to eat dairy, eat full fat options—cream,

yoghurt, butter and cheeses. Avoid milk due to high lactose content. (When you check out what some high level athletes eat in a later chapter, you will observe a high level of heavy whipping cream in their diet.)

Natural herbs and spices are fine as long as there's no added sugar or MSG.

So you see there is plenty to choose from. It is not restrictive and most diets that lean towards eating healthy, natural foods will contain a very similar list.

I advise you to chart your carbohydrates daily in the early days as so many foods do contain carbohydrates; you will be surprised how easily it is to go above 300g very quickly (even when you thought you were cutting back!).

There are plenty of free tools to help you do this like http://www.myfitnesspal.com or http://keto-calculator.ankerl .com/

*** ***

Here is the list of the NOT "allowed" foods:

Do Not Eat:

Most things in a wrapper! Avoid highly processed foods. Go for natural foods.

Avoid high carbohydrate foods like breads, pastas, and rice. Avoid breakfast cereals (including muesli and granola), sandwiches, sports gels, sugary snacks, bagels, cookies, cakes, sweets, and ice cream.

Avoid all flours from grains—wheat flour, corn flour, rye flour, barley flour, pea flour, rice flour, and all forms of bread and all grains—wheat, oats, barley, rye, amaranth, quinoa and teff.

Avoid beans, legumes (no lentils, chickpeas or beans, though a small amount of green beans and peas may be allowed once you are keto-adapted). Peanuts are also a legume (not a nut) and should be avoided.

Avoid corn products like popcorn, polenta and maize. No couscous, millet or buckwheat, no cakes or confectionery.

No sugary drinks like Coca Cola, Fanta, sugary milkshakes or fruit juice. No lite, zero or diet drinks of any description. No beer or cider.

Avoid most fruits as they contain too much sugar. But you may eat a small amount of blueberries, raspberries and strawberries on occasion.

As stated above, be careful with dairy. Eliminate it for a month then re-introduce gradually and see how you feel. It can be a good source of fat if your body can tolerate it. However, only have full-fat options.

Avoid commercial cheese spreads, coffee creamers commercial almond milk, condensed milk, anything fat-free or skimmed and soymilk and rice milk.

Avoid margarine, vegetable oils, seed oils, commercial marinades or salad dressings.

Avoid sweets, artificial sweeteners (aspartame, acesulfame K, saccharin, sucralose, splenda), syrups, sugar, dried fruit, agave anything and cordials.

Instead of noticing all the things you can't eat, focus on the list of all the things you can eat. Acknowledge that you will never be hungry. There is plenty to eat and you are not restricting calories.

***

Analysis Of My Pre-Post Keto Diet and Macros So Far

I urge you to start by charting a "normal" day for you before you start the ketogenic diet so you see where you are coming from. Track your current diet and macros (fat, carbohydrate and protein) so you can see your current baseline.

This will help you plan your week ahead.

Remember you are aiming for your calories to come from 70-75% fat, 5%-10% carbohydrate and 20% protein. It may take a week or so to get this dialled in.

If you are endeavouring to get into ketosis, you are aiming to stay between 25g and 50g carbs for the day initially.

To give you an idea from my experience, a normal diet for me pre-ketogenic contained 235g of carbohydrate!

This diet was traditionally "healthy" from Western point of view but still way over the ketogenic carbohydrate level. And I need to point out that this was without any gels or sports drinks that I would certainly have taken on a 2-hour+ cycle. So on those days I would be easily over 300g of carbohydrate.

A typical pre-ketogenic day for me consisted of cereal/oatmeal, banana and coffee for breakfast, ham salad sandwich for lunch, snacks might be 3-4 pieces of fruit, a handful of nuts and cheese and crackers. Maybe a juice or smoothie and plenty of water. Dinner was chicken or fish, vegetables and rice or pasta. Maybe a glass of wine and a couple of pieces of chocolate.

So pretty healthy—no sweets, desserts, takeaways, and minimal processed food. But there were still far too many carbohydrates to achieve ketogenic heaven.

Now a typical day would be bacon and poached eggs on spinach for breakfast, tuna and salad for lunch, chicken or fish with vegetables for dinner.

Snacks—a handful of nuts, sliced avocado, some yoghurt or a couple of pieces of dark chocolate.

I add plenty of butter to my vegetables, coconut oil to my salads and full cream to my coffee.

Now my carbohydrate level is 52 grams, so a big improvement but there is still work to be done.

Interestingly, I was always a massive snacker. Now I rarely feel the need to snack.

Charlotte Campbell Pre/Post Ketogenic Diet Macros

	Pre-Keto	Pre %	Post-Keto	Target (g)	Current %	Target (%)
Fat	90g	40%	139g	156g	68%	70%
Protein	74g	15%	93g	100g	20%	20%
Carbs	235g	45%	52g	25-50g	12%	10%

Note: To convert grams into calories:
Grams of fat x 9
Grams of protein and carbs x 4

I still need to increase my fat intake even more. Interestingly, I have increased my fat intake from 40% to 68% and I have lost 3 kg by doing so during the initial 4 weeks and 4% body fat. I am very pleased with that.

Who would have thought?

I am almost at the initial target percentages and plan to stay there for another 4 weeks. Then I will tweak it again to 80% fat content and see what happens.

My experience on this diet has been very positive. I have been surprised how easy it was actually. Occasionally, if I meet friends for coffee and they are ordering croissants or pastries with their coffee, I feel a pang of temptation (but I have not succumbed)!

This is still not perfect and there is more tweaking to do. I would like to get my carbs down below 40g. I probably eat too many nuts when I do choose to have a snack and occasionally have a few more squares of dark chocolate in the evening instead of just the 2 squares I have allowed myself.

Most of it is habit rather than hunger. I have not been hungry or felt deprived (well, except maybe when the smell of those fresh croissants came to my table...).

As far as my training goes, I am currently in a low intensity base phase, doing 1-2 hour sessions at a low heart rate, so I have not felt the need for any sports drinks or gels as yet. But in another 4 weeks, when I increase the intensity of training again, I will be definitely keto-adapted and it should be a lot easier to drink water only for the 2-3 hour sessions.

I am definitely in ketosis, but it can take anywhere from 6-12 weeks to build the right metabolic enzymes, fat-burning pathways and "machinery" to be certain of prioritizing burning fat as fuel.

Pretty much any shade of pink means you are in ketosis. Beige means you are not in ketosis. It does not matter if your shade of pink does not match your friend's shade of pink. Everyone will be different.

Ketostix are just a guide. They are fallible and there can be different reasons for false positives and negatives. So use this tool if you find it helpful but do not obsess about it.

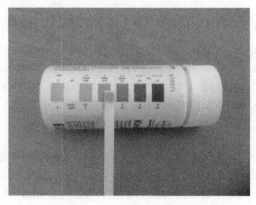

Charlotte Campbell Ketostix result

It is generally helpful in the beginning to get confirmation that the changes you are making are working. Many people who are fully keto-adapted get negative readings because their body is efficiently using all their ketones for fuel so there are no extra ketones to be excreted.

There are other indicators, of course, like body weight, body fat %, energy levels, appetite levels, performance levels, sleep patterns, GI distress levels, IBS, acne and so on. So track a few indicators that make sense for you.

But if you are ingesting 25-50g per day, you will be in ketosis.

Remember there are times when you may be able to ingest 100g carbohydrates and still be in ketosis if you have a large muscle mass, do a ton of exercise, and have a bigger body frame. But do not assume this will be you. Stay strict at first, get the fundamentals right before you start go off-piste!

Step-by Step Guide To Getting Started

Sometimes it can be difficult to absorb all the information and put it together in a logical way that makes sense. So I have tried to do that here in case you are at the beginning of your keto journey and feeling a bit overwhelmed.

Step1

Chart your normal macros on your pre-ketogenic diet to see where you are now. Take your baseline measurements of whatever you want to track: body weight, body fat%, how many gels you require during a 3-hour ride at 200W etc.

Step 2

Write your food plan for the week of what you will actually eat—breakfast, lunch, dinner and snacks.

Step 3

Shop for your ketogenic diet and prepare some meals ahead if possible.

Step 4

Clear your week for a stable or easier training week just in case.

Step 5

Be aware that your body will be going through a massive adjustment. The first 2-4 days, you may have "hunger pangs"(though you won't actually be hungry), sugar cravings or "keto flu".

So plan for this by getting plenty of sunshine and plenty of sleep. Add electrolytes to your diet (sodium, potassium and magnesium). Drink plenty of water.

Step 6

Test your ketone levels. Daily at first, later you will not need to at all. Also record your subjective results of how you are feeling and objective measures.

Step 7

Keep exercising at low intensity. Aerobic exercise (especially in a fasted state) will help you become fat-adapted sooner.

*** ***

You have all the allowed foods so be creative with what you can eat. Make sure you find some things you like or you won't keep it up. At no point should you feel deprived or hungry.

In a later chapter, I will give you some actual daily food plans of some famous ketogenic endurance athletes and tell you what they actually eat during a typical day so you can see how they put together the list of allowed foods and produce incredible endurance performances on that.

This is a critical chapter for endurance athletes and one that most books on the ketogenic diet do not even touch upon.

As athletes, this chapter is vital to getting athletic success to compliment your dietary success. You cannot have one without the other.

For most of the population, whose exercise consists of something between "nothing" and "walking the dog for 20 minutes twice a day", the ability to pump out huge exercise sessions whilst they adapt to a ketogenic diet is not a major concern.

They can manage to continue their normal life and activities quite easily. But what about for us athletes who train at intensity, high volume and always have a race coming up?

The three biggest fears athletes have when they are considering the ketogenic diet (or any change in diet) are:

1. Will it take much time to get used to it and prepare food?
2. Will I get a dip in performance initially?
3. Will I spend most of my day hungry?

This is totally understandable and correct training methods are what this chapter will focus on…

How To Ensure The Ketogenic Diet Enhances Your Training Successfully

Logically you know that if you have been doing one thing for many years, to make a sudden change can upset the body's equilibrium for a few weeks until it recalibrates.

Then there is a bit of mental energy spent getting used to the new program.

Even though you may understand or hope that the change will make a great improvement to your results *long term*, you often cannot stand to face the *short-term* loss of strength or loss of performance required to get there so you just keep doing what you have always done.

BUT, AS EINSTEIN SAID, "IF YOU DO WHAT YOU'VE ALWAYS DONE, YOU WILL GET WHAT YOU'VE ALWAYS GOT."

So, if you know your diet is sub-standard, full of processed foods packed with chemicals, preservatives and e-numbers, almost ANY change in diet to one based on natural foods will boost your results.

It does not matter whether it is Paleo, vegan or a fruit juice diet!

Let's address these 3 biggest fears head on because you may be thinking the same things:

1. **Will it take much time to get used to it and prepare food?**

   Yes, it will take some time to get used to it. Not long though.

   Most athletes report that after 2 weeks they are fine. To be honest it will depend a lot on what your current diet is. If you currently eat a ton of processed food and take-aways, you will no doubt suffer sugar cravings for a few days.

You will also have to learn to shop in a completely different aisle. Maybe you spend a lot of time in the pasta, bread and cookie aisle. You will need to discover the fresh meat, fish and vegetable sections.

Preparing food can be as easy as making scrambled eggs in 5 minutes or making up a large chicken and vegetable dish for the week. It is up to you.

As always, for maximum efficiency, I recommend you make a big batch of a couple of dishes on a Sunday then your meals are prepared for the week well in advance so no brain work or thought is required every night to work out what to eat.

EFFICIENCY AND TIME MANAGEMENT ARE KEY FOR ANYTHING NEW TO WORK

Initially you may have the feeling of "Groan—now I have to think before I eat instead of grabbing my favorite items whenever I feel hungry."

Yes, this will be the case with every diet. Make sure you have some healthy snacks on hand so if you are desperate to graze, you can reach for something that does not pollute your body with sugar. Luckily, the ketogenic diet has plenty to eat, most of which is readily available everywhere so really this is a very minor concern.

2. Will I get a dip in performance initially?

Some athletes experience what is called "keto flu" for 1-2 weeks after starting the ketogenic diet. This is largely due to the drop in blood sugar levels, which also drops the sodium levels in your blood so you may feel tired and blurry for a few days.

This is easily remedied by adding electrolytes to your diet. Add sodium, potassium and magnesium and this will help you avoid these symptoms.

I would not recommend any drastic change in diet 4 weeks prior to a race or during an intense training block. But this does not mean waiting until the off-season. If you are in a stable, manageable training phase, you may start this diet.

Some athletes experience no "keto flu" at all if they had good diets to begin with. For example, many of the people who switch from Paleo find they have 80% of the diet dialled in anyway. If they switch to a ketogenic diet, they are simply making small tweaks.

For everyone else, add some electrolytes and you should avoid "keto flu" as well.

3. Will I spend most of my day hungry?

One of the best things about the ketogenic diet (and why it works so well for athletes) is that there is no calorie restriction.

Yay! You can eat as much as you want. You are simply changing the ratio of carbs, protein and fat you ingest. You can have snacks during the day and still eat big meals if you want to.

What tends to happen is that after 2-4 weeks, you will find that you rarely feel like snacking as you eat nutrient-rich foods and due to eating a large proportion of fat you will not get hungry.

Successful Training Principles That Will Supercharge Your Results On The Ketogenic Diet

The ketogenic diet is aimed at activating the fat-burning mechanisms of our body and reducing reliance on using glucose as the primary fuel source.

Logically then, your training program should support that same aim to burn fat, not sugar, as your fuel source in order to accelerate your results.

Great results on the ketogenic diet come from:

1. Reducing the amount of glucose on hand in the body for the body to use. The body will use whatever is most readily available—carbohydrate, fat or protein.

   If there is glucose around in the blood stream, the body will use that first as too much sugar is toxic in the body so it will always metabolize this first.

2. Allowing the body to rebuild its "machinery" to burn fat for energy easily. The more you reduce glucose, the more the body will increase its level of fat-burning enzymes and fat-burning pathways.

   So if you optimize your training to be aerobic in nature, you will accelerate the rate at which your body's fat-burning capacity improves.

   If you keep "slipping up" in the early days, either by gorging on sugar or by doing predominantly anaerobic training, the body will quickly flip back to sugar-burning mechanisms and it will take so much longer to become fat-adapted.

   However, if you are strict in the beginning, and your training (aerobic training to encourage fat burning) complements your diet (eat higher proportion of fat to encourage fat burning), your fat-burning mechanisms will be improved, optimized and work efficiently.

Once you are fat-adapted and have built your metabolic machinery and fat-burning pathways, you are allowed to have some extra carbohydrate if necessary during an Ironman or a 100 mile ultra, as your body can instantly switch back to fat burning the next day. It has built the required tools.

Until then, stay strict!

Aerobic training (means with oxygen) is done at a pace at which you can easily hold a conversation.

Anaerobic training (means without oxygen) is done with intensity so you are puffing and panting.

Traditional Methods of Fuelling

Let's look at the traditional way most endurance athletes get fuel during exercise. You have been taught to eat predominantly carbohydrate as an athlete. You may also have been encouraged to eat tons more carbohydrate the day before an event to fill up your glycogen stores to the maximum level.

However, no matter what you do, the body can only store 1800-2200 calories of carbohydrates in the form of glycogen in the liver. This is a massive limitation in your triathlon races (or any endurance event).

One of the most common reasons athletes must pull out of a race is gastric distress due to gulping down too many gels and slurping too many sports drinks.

Once that glycogen supply has gone (usually 1-2hours exercise), your body literally stops. You "bonk". The gas tank is empty. With all the greatest will in the world you cannot continue unless you take on more carbohydrate. Hence the proliferation of gels, bars and sports drinks.

But even if you re-fuel at 200-600 calories per hour, which is all the stomach can handle, you will run out of glycogen in a longer event or at the very least be last seen puking in a bush as your stomach rejects the excessive gels you have to ingest.

You will experience "bonking" where you literally run out of energy despite the fact that your body may(!) be carrying excess fat (and therefore has access to unlimited energy but it just does not have the pathways and enzymes to turn this into energy yet!).

Quite simply, if your exercise is anaerobic, this limited supply of glycogen plus whatever amount of gels your stomach can handle is your primary energy source.

However, is it not ridiculous that you are carrying around an almost endless supply of energy (fat) but you cannot access it easily?

1lb of fat used during aerobic exercise contains 4000 calories. Even if you are a lean 5% body fat athlete, your available fat (if you weight 10.7st) is 7.5lb. This can keep you going for several hundred miles. You have access to 30,000 available calories for energy (instead of just 2000 calories stored as glycogen in the liver).

If you are a "normal" athlete (at the same 10.7st) with 15% body fat, you have access to 90,000 available calories for energy!

THE TRICK TO ACCESSING THIS ALMOST UNLIMITED ENERGY SOURCE IS THAT *YOU MUST REMAIN AEROBIC WHILST AT HIGHER SPEEDS*

Here is what to do:

Principle 1: Improve Your Aerobic Efficiency

Correct aerobic training is done at a pace at which you can still easily hold a conversation. This encourages fat-burning mechanisms and complements a true ketogenic diet.

Many Type A triathletes, cyclists and runners actually skip this important aerobic training and go straight into the hard stuff because they feel they are not improving in fitness quick enough at lower intensities.

They never do "easy" training thinking it is a "waste of time". Do you know anyone like this?

Most triathletes either do high intensity training or moderate-hard cardio training and always train in the sugar-burning zone.

Now, do not get me wrong! I am not saying you should never train at high intensity. I LOVE high intensity. But FIRST you must build an efficient machine that runs on efficient fuel.

THEN *once* you have an efficient engine, you can add on high intensity, resistance work and speed work as you please.

There are two good ways to be sure you are training in your aerobic zone:

1. Strap on a heart rate monitor and do not exercise more than 180-your age.

Or

2. Train only at the exercise intensity that you can comfortably breathe through your nose.

This happens to be about the same as your desired heart rate (180-your age).

This way of training encourages an efficient exchange of oxygen and maintains an aerobic pace. It also encourages primarily fat burning.

Obviously, this requires discipline. There is always the temptation to do this for 15 minutes then get bored and ramp it up so you "feel like you've had a good workout".

This is a mistake as it will switch you straight over into sugar burning as the fuel source and you will take forever to become a fat-burning machine.

Do you train in the black hole?

Most triathletes train in the "black hole". This is a common mistake that many endurance athletes make where they train at intensity that is not high intensity enough to be in the anaerobic zone, but it is too high intensity to be in the aerobic zone.

It basically achieves nothing except glucose burning, oxidative damage and an increase in free radicals in the body. Of course, training in "no man's land" will still get you fit.

But at what cost?

It will not get you fitter than training smart. Plus you will get accelerated ageing, higher likelihood of disease and less longevity as an athlete.

Structure your training so you do not train in the "black hole".

Principle 2: Ditch Chronic Cardio

It is very important for your long-term health not to spend much time in the "black hole".

As triathletes, runners or cyclists, we tend to do a lot of mileage. Some of this is essential.

However, a lot of it is done without much thought towards "Can this be done better and more efficiently?"

Ask the questions, "How can I do this better?" and, "How can I get more results with less time?"

Rather than:

"How can I fit in more mileage?"

There is a frightening amount of research and information[50] from the scientific and medical community already that shows that chronic cardio training is bad for your heart, causing scarring of the arteries and chronic inflammation in the body.

Even more scary is the fact that a number of high profile athletes have either dropped dead suddenly or had heart issues at an early age.

I do not want to spend too long on this but it is important so I will give you some resources you can dive into this deeper if you wish to.

Cardiologist Dr. James O'Keefe has done a lot of research into this. Watch his TED talk here[51].

The first recorded case of heart problems associated with long distance exercise occurred in 490BC. Phidippides, a professional long distance runner in 5th century BC, was the first recorded case of a very fit athlete dropping dead suddenly.

Phidippides was asked by the Athenian generals to run 140 miles to Sparta to ask for help re an impending Persian invasion. He did so (it took him 36 hours). Phidippides then ran back to Athens (another 140 miles!) with their message.

He then immediately fought in the battle of Marathon as a soldier.

He was then asked to run 26 miles (3 hours) from Marathon to Athens to proclaim the victory over the Persians, after which he collapsed and died (aged 40 years old). He was an accomplished long distance runner. A 3-hour run was not unusual for him. It is likely he developed some scarring on the heart over time and cardiomyopathy.

In another case, most of you have probably read the excellent book by Christopher McDougall, *Born to Run*, describing the story of Micah True, a legendary long distance runner (the mythic Caballo Blanco). He would regularly run 100 miles in a day.

He died suddenly while on a routine 12-mile training run March 27, 2012 aged 58 years old. On autopsy, it was found his heart was enlarged with scar tissue. He had the same pathology found in extreme ultra-athletes—cardiomyopathy, a condition caused by chronic excessive endurance exercise. It is now called "Phidippides cardiomyopathy".

Sadly, there are countless others. Experienced marathoner Ryan Shay[52] (aged 28) and Ironman triathlete Steve Larsen[53] (aged 39) both died suddenly due to cardiac arrest.

Greg Welch[54], the only triathlete in the world to win world titles in Ironman, long distance triathlon, Olympic distance triathlon and duathlon suffered ventricular tachycardia and needed nine open-heart surgeries from 2001 until 2003 (aged 37-39).

Emma Carney[55], Australian professional triathlete and twice World Triathlon Champion, suffered a cardiac arrest in 2004 (aged 33), was diagnosed with ventricular tachycardia (electrical abnormality in the heart) and had to have a pacemaker fitted for life.

These cases are frightening! And what about all the ones we have not heard about?

But this is not intended to scare you off, it is simply to highlight the need to train smarter and be aware of what impact your training is having so you can avoid damaging your body (when you are thinking you are improving your health).

For instance, at the end of a marathon or Ironman triathlon, we all have micro-tears of the heart muscle. This is not usually a problem as long as we take sufficient rest afterwards.

A few days later, these micro tears will heal. But what if we do this over and over again without sufficient rest? The heart chambers become hard, scarred and thickened. The risk of atrial fibrillation increases five-fold.

Wait a second; isn't exercise supposed to add years to my life?

Please note: running and exercise are NOT bad for you.

(I still train 5-6 days a week and compete in triathlons. But I certainly am much more aware of the need for recovery and planning out specific training blocks with a specific purpose rather than my old view of "train as hard as possible all the time" and "recovery is for wimps".)

If you are intelligent as to *how* you train, you will ensure your long-term health is looked after plus perform a lot better in the short term with much less stress on your body.

What does this mean?

It means you should allow your body to do some regular, easy training as well as the intense stuff. After an intense workout or training block, allow sufficient rest.

The problem with "black hole" training is that the "easy days" are never really easy (as you push too hard) and the hard days are never truly hard as you are too fatigued from previous sessions and do not take enough rest to push into the higher zones on your "hard" day.

You end up doing chronic cardio in "no man's land" (damaging for the heart) and not getting the fitness changes you deserve.

If you never feel rested, this is also a problem! I know; I have been there in the past!

Training, work, family, social commitments, committee meetings, bills, travel, pressure and the list goes on.

Look at your lifestyle.
Look at your diet.
Look at your training schedule.

Could you achieve more with less training?
Do you need any supplements?
Do you need to meditate?
Do you need to do yoga or tai chi or simply go to bed 30 minutes earlier?

Consider heart rate variability training[56], which can help monitor how well your body has recovered after training sessions. It can be a useful tool if you often get injured or sick or feel over trained.

Whether you decide to use one of these tools or just go on

intuition and self-awareness, you should only do MAX intensity sessions when you are rested and really feel up for it.

Do not do high intensity training when you feel physically sore from a previous session or if you are mentally tired. Take another day's rest or do an easy aerobic session. You WILL get better results.

Principle 3: Train Smart: Periodization

You need to know what the aim of each training session is and why.

Plan this out roughly in advance along with your key races or key goals for the year ahead. But allow yourself some flex within that. Blasting ahead with a tough session just because it is in your planner but you do not feel 100% recovered is not smart. As you become a better athlete, learn to listen to your body more.

If you have a hard session planned but you are still sore from a previous session or fatigued and stressed from work, you would be foolish to do the scheduled hard session. You will not be able to get to the right intensity and you will be training in no man's land or be unable to maintain good form and risk injury.

If you are doing an easy session, practice the discipline to stay easy (do not creep up into "no mans land" of "moderately difficult" just because you feel you could go faster!).

The easy session is there for a reason. It is important to do easy sessions in base training to improve your aerobic efficiency and fat-burning pathways. It is important to do easy sessions for recovery from hard training blocks during your strength or speed training phases.

It has immense training benefits.

Strap a heart rate monitor on to make sure you stay in the right zone. Measure your aerobic capacity and track improvements once a month (see MAF test below).

By the way, if you are a triathlete or are thinking of trying a triathlon, you are welcome to join our Free 5-Day Triathlon Accelerator Course (http://www.triathlon-hacks.com/free-course).

Principle 4: Test and Measure Your Aerobic Capacity: MAF TEST (Maximum aerobic function)

Dr. Phil Maffetone[57] has been coaching, training and researching this topic for over 40 years.

His view:

DO YOU WANT SPEED? THEN SLOW DOWN!
GO SLOW TO GO FAST

Low intensity does not mean you will go slow for ever! It means creating fat-burning pathways that will make you faster over time.

Why do some people puff and pant when running at 8-minute miles while elite runners can comfortably chat and laugh when running easy at 6-minute miles?

It is due to improved aerobic capacity. This is the ability to run faster *at your aerobic capacity.*

Here is an example from an athlete who worked closely with Dr. Maffetone:

Mike Pigg was an elite triathlete who was famous for the traditional "go hard or go home" triathlete mentality. He was considered one of the hardest-working athletes in the sport.

He dominated the short-course triathlon scene from the late 1980s to the mid 1990s, with an astonishing thirty wins in the USA Triathlon Series. Unsurprisingly, he suffered burnout and injury and was not getting the results he wanted for the pain he was putting into hard training sessions and he was on the verge of quitting.

He sought out Dr. Phil Maffetone. Dr. Maffetone advised him to train below heart rate 155bpm. Mike, who was already super fit and used to training hard, found this almost impossible! He found himself walking up hills he could easily run up just to maintain this low heart rate.

However, he was determined to get success and persisted despite his reservations. He was still sceptical that this would work but he sometimes cycled with Mark Allen (who also worked with Phil Maffetone). Mike noticed that Mark could keep his heart rate 10-15bpm lower than him and always had abundant energy whereas Mike was sucking down extra gels all the time just to keep going.

Mike began to change his diet, reduce carbohydrates and increase protein and fat. After five months of loyal, consistent training (below 155bpm), he started to see results.

Mike recalled a 65-mile ride he did regularly. He would usually complete it in 4 hours, arriving exhausted and hungry at an average heart rate of 165bpm.

Within 5 months of Maffetone training, he was shocked to find he could now do the same 65-mile ride in 3 hours at 155bpm. Plus he could go straight out for a 10-mile run on arrival and did not feel hungry.

OK- he was fitter at lower intensities but what about racing?

The results translated into faster race pace.

Mike had not done any high intensity race pace sessions and lacked confidence for racing. He was booked on the first race of the season in Australia at the Surfers Paradise International Triathlon and did not want to go. He thought he would come last as he had done no speed work in months and wanted to pull out. However, he told himself to just "get round" and have a good time.

To his surprise, he won the race!

He was sold!

Mike stresses that this doesn't mean that endurance athletes can't train anaerobically, performing hard interval sessions. But this approach to developing speed is not a priority.

Instead, developing aerobic speed, where you can run much faster with the same effort compared to weeks and months earlier, is the priority.

This not only provides significant speed during training and racing, but it's accomplished with much less stress, so the risk of injury and overtraining is greatly reduced.

Despite this, many endurance athletes expend significant time and energy on intensely hard anaerobic workouts, often neglecting or impairing the aerobic system in the process.

This is not smart training. In a one-hour event, 98% of your endurance energy is derived from the aerobic system; in a two-hour event, 99% is derived from the aerobic system.

DOES IT MAKE SENSE TO SPEND SO MANY HOURS A WEEK ON ANAEROBIC WORK WHEN 99% OF YOUR RACE ENERGY COMES FROM THE AEROBIC SYSTEM?

Instead, it's best to first derive your endurance speed from aerobic training, and then, as time and energy permits, to add spurts of anaerobic training.

Mark Allen, as we discussed, also worked with the Dr. Maffetone method. Allen was previously at the stage of burnout and injury. Maffetone diagnosed aerobic deficiency and anaerobic excess.

Dr. Maffetone suggested he trained <150bpm. Mark Allen, a six-time Ironman champion, took time off from racing to train by the MAF method.

At the beginning of his aerobic training period, it was difficult for him. He was jogging 12-minute miles!

Crazy for an elite athlete! Slowly but surely, his speed began to increase, and as his aerobic efficiency improved, he got back down to his usual training speed. Only this time he was running aerobically at that speed.

Allen stopped getting injured and came back to win 6 more World Champion Triathlon titles in Kona.

Incredible!

What works for these super athletes will work for us! Even they had to go back and start from scratch in order to move forward.

Even the best athletes (actually, especially the best) do the majority of their training at an aerobic heart rate. They only do one or two days of anaerobic training a week.

That is the basic MAF recommendation. If the majority of your training is anaerobic, getting injured won't be a matter of luck; it'll be a matter of time.

But if you have a good base, one or two anaerobic days a week will keep you strong and powerful. However, be sure to spend a couple of months a year (the winter is the best time) doing nothing but slow, aerobic training.

What about high intensity training?

Do NOT skip the base training phase.

Building your aerobic engine and fat-burning capabilities requires that you hold yourself back, as difficult as that may be to do.

This will ensure you can do more and go faster within your aerobic zone and activate your fat-burning pathways (unlimited energy).

Do 8 weeks of aerobic training *without* adding in strength or speed work. If you get a cold, get sick or injured, the 8-week period starts again. This period will take as long as it takes.

Some people might take 8 weeks, others may take 5 months!

If you are getting NO improvements, do not throw it out the window. Remember Mike Pigg and Mark Allen winning their subsequent events! Instead, slow down *even more* and start the 8-week timeline again.

Do no high intensity or interval training until you have completed 8 weeks base training with aerobic improvements and no illness or injury.

When you commence high intensity training, do not do it constantly for 8 weeks. Instead only do it for a 2-3 week block then allow recovery. Never do it for more than 4 weeks straight without recovery.

Take-aways so far:

Do no blended workouts. Do not do aerobic training with sprints or strength work at the end.

Do base training first for at least 8 weeks.

If you are doing strength training, lift heavy, do low reps then go home. Do not do high reps of light weights and turn it into an aerobic session[58].

If you are doing an easy session, make sure it is at heart rate below 180-your age and do not let your heart rate drift up.

If you are doing high intensity, go hard then allow time to recover. Never do high intensity for more than 2-3 weeks without allowing sufficient recovery.

What shall I do in the off-season?

Have a rest! Complete rest for 4 weeks is ideal. You can be active but do not train, do not read books about training, do not think about training. Move your body in different ways. Go ice-skating, kick a ball around, go hiking, do yoga.

After this complete break, start base training. Do this for at least 8 weeks every year. Go back to these fundamentals. Do nothing but slow, aerobic training.

Review your season. What were your weaknesses? Plan to work on those.

You may need:

- a gait analysis to improve your running technique
- some massage sessions to clear knots that have built up in your muscles
- yoga to finally improve your flexibility
- some personal training sessions in the gym to strengthen your core or get coaching on your deadlift

What is the MAF method?

Dr. Phil Maffetone uses the 180 formula[59]: **180-your age.**

So if you are 30 years old, all your aerobic training is done below a heart rate of 180-30=150bpm. This will help you build an efficient aerobic base. Training above this heart rate will kick in the anaerobic system and switch your fuel source from predominantly fat to predominantly sugar.

Is this simple? Yes

Is it easy? No

IT IS THE HARDEST THING
IN THE WORLD TO SLOW DOWN

The question is do you want to improve as an athlete?

Many athletes do a lot of training that has absolutely no benefit to their health or their performance. This is wasted time.

If you train at a heart rate too high for aerobic changes and too low for productive speed or strength improvements, you are burning sugar and placing unnecessary work on your heart.

Let's assume you are 40 years old and can normally run at 8-minute miles. But on the Maffetone method, you need to stay under 140bpm. Now you can only run at 11-minute miles while maintaining 140bpm. It means you are not aerobically efficient.

However, keep training this way and over several weeks you will notice you can soon run at 10-minute miles whilst below 140bpm, then 9-minute miles whilst below 140bpm, then 8-minute miles whilst below 140bpm and beyond.

Being able to run the same speed as before at an "easy " heart rate and using fat (instead of sugar) as your unlimited fuel source is a smart way to train.

Bike example:

Stay below heart rate140bpm. Perhaps you can only push 170W for 30 minutes without your heart rate shooting up. Over a period of weeks you will be able to achieve 210W, then 250W, then 270W at this same heart rate of 140bpm.

You are building the metabolic machinery to access ketones for fuel. If you do not have the patience to do the work, you will still be a sugar burner and your heart rate will go through the roof.

However, if you can perform more work at a lower heart rate, by the time you get to a race you will be unstoppable.

What is the MAF test?

A very important factor to help us stay on track with any diet or program is measuring and tracking your results. This provides motivation when you see that you are improving, especially if you are sceptical! Plus it allows you to tweak and improve things early if you are not progressing as expected.

The MAF Test[60] can be done with any cardio exercise to measure improvements in aerobic efficiency.

The test:

Workout (swim, jog or cycle) at your maximum *aerobic* heart rate (180-your age). Record the time it takes you to cover a certain distance.

Perform this same distance test once a month to ensure that each time you are faster over the same distance at the same heart rate. This means your aerobic system is developing and you're burning more fat, enabling you to do more work with the same effort.

Dr. Steve Phinney[61] has done a ton of research into athletic performance and low carb diet. In one study with runners and rowers, some on a low carb diet, some on a traditional high carb diet, he found the low carb group burned more fat than previously thought possible. He realized that once you become fat-adapted, you will also burn more fat at higher intensities.

Add strength training

Strength training is essential in endurance sports. Many neglect it completely, which is a mistake. If you neglect it due to "lack of time" this is false economy as it usually takes less than 30 minutes and will give you far greater results than going out for another 2-hour bike ride.

Putting your muscle under load stimulates positive hormonal adaptations and helps preserve good technique and maximal power production during endurance workouts. Improved strength is essential to help you maintain good form towards the end of an event when everyone else is fatiguing.

The main reason many endurance athletes do not see great results from strength training is that they do not do it properly. It is common for endurance athletes to turn their strength session into yet another cardio session by doing low weights and high repetitions.

It looks something like this: Hold 2kg dumbbells and do 3 sets of 25 reps.

This is a complete waste of time and a big mistake.

If you decide to do strength workout then do a strength workout. Do not turn it into a cardio workout.

Lift the heaviest weight you can lift 5 times. Concentrate on good form. When you fatigue and either lose form or cannot complete 5 reps, you stop, change the exercise or go home.

Do not be tempted to reduce the weight to continue as this then turns it into a cardio session. So if you are doing squats with 70 kg on your back then you fatigue, do not drop the weight to 50kg and continue.

By the way, if you are over 40 years old (either gender), strength training is even more important to maintain muscle mass and good hormonal function. Plus, as a bonus, strength training has a profound anti-ageing effect.

Endurance athletes *need* to be strong. If you hit a hill at mile 16, you need sufficient power to get over the hill. You will need to recruit more muscle fibers. These are recruited in maximal gym workouts.

If there are 3 hills in a race and you have done your strength training, you are likely to see your power look like this:

First hill: 100% maximum power
Second hill: 95% maximum power
Third hill: 92% maximum power.

If you avoided strength training and are a sugar burner, you will see something like this:

First hill: 100% maximum power
Second hill: 89% maximum power
Third hill: 63% maximum power

When strength training, be sure to focus on large muscle group, compound exercises. The most relevant exercises include squats, deadlifts, push-ups, chin ups, and lunges.

Add high intensity training

June 2005, Martin Gibala of MacMaster University[63] reported that 6 minutes of pure, hard exercise 3 times a week was just as effective as 1 hour of moderate daily activity.

Changes that were thought to require hours of training per week were achieved with 4-7 bursts of 30-second all-out (250%VO2max) stationary cycling with 4 minutes recovery between each one.

This was repeated 3-times a week for just 2 weeks.Total on-bike time over 2 weeks was just 15 minutes.

Most relevant to us, their endurance capacity almost doubled from 26 minutes to 51 minutes! This is incredible!

Their leg muscles showed 38% increase in endurance enzymes.

The control group who were active (jogging, cycling or aerobics) showed no changes.

Was it a fluke?

The test was repeated and this time the test was a 30km(18.6 miles) cycling test.

The test group did the same 30-second burst protocol

above. The control group this time did moderate intensity 60-90 minutes at 60% VO2max. Both groups worked out 3 times a week.

The results were almost identical as the test above.

Conclusion: Do not do exactly the same protocol of 60 minutes' moderate intensity work every day.

Mix it up.

When it is time to go hard, go short and hard. Then allow recovery. When it is time to go easy, make sure you have the discipline to go easy.

Do not do mid range "no man's land" training.

IT IS NOT NECESSARY TO SPEND HOURS DOING MEDIOCRE TRAINING

Instead understand what gives you the better results in the shortest period of time and do that. Then get on with enjoying the rest of your life.

Some examples of elite endurance athletes following these training principles

Sami Inkinen[62] is a super successful triathlete. He is a serial entrepreneur running a huge company of over 300 people. He has won Wildflower 70.3 and finishes sub 9-hours at Kona.

He believes the high volume chronic cardio 25-30 hours a week typical Ironman program is not necessary. He only trains 10-12 hours a week.

He has a demanding job and family commitments to fit in. He attributes his success to:

- Strict adherence to recovery between sessions

- Short, high intensity exercise (after established aerobic baseline) and

- Eating a high-fat low-carb diet (ketogenic)

His philosophy is that if he is not fully recovered from a previous workout, he won't benefit from this workout, so he takes another rest day. He does not skip on sleep to train. Sleep is massively important for recovery.

Sami advises forgetting gels and sugary drinks for post workout re-fuelling. His post workout re-fuelling meal includes protein and salad.

Brian Mackenzie[63], founder of Cross Fit Endurance, produces 100-mile runners on less than 30 miles total running per week. (This is vastly different to traditional running of 80-100 miles a week, which is normal for long distance runners.)

After developing a good baseline, Mackenzie trains his runners on a lot of high intensity work. He also shares the view discussed above that once you lose form or your heart rate does not recover swiftly between intervals you go home. Session over.

For instance, in Tabata training he says if your heart rate does not return to 120 within 2 minutes the workout is over.

Similarities:

All these pro and elite athletes prioritize recovery. Yes, they train hard—when their bodies are ready (and not before). They limit the amount of training hours and get incredible results!

More Advanced Workout Considerations

What we have discussed here are the guiding principles that

you can build your training plan from. It is impossible to give one training plan as it is different for sprint triathletes versus Ironman athletes. It is also different depending on your current fitness levels.

Do not over-complicate it. Keep it as simple as possible and just make a start. Maybe you do get everything right straight away, maybe you don't.

It does not matter as long as you are moving towards a better, healthier and more productive way of eating and training that takes less time, is more enjoyable and will help you become a better athlete.

There will be times in your training when you need to make tweaks depending on your training or racing needs.

Once you adapt to using fat for fuel, the body does not stop storing glycogen. It still refuels its glycogen stores. The ketogenic way of eating and training means your body now has a glycogen sparing effect. You will still use some glycogen in a race, you will just be able to prioritize and access fat for energy as well.

Greg McMillan supports this view. The key aims of the long, slow aerobic training are to increase your ability to burn fat, to train the mind to keep going when you feel fatigued and to train the body to exercise with low blood glucose levels and still be able to function well.

When you have adapted to this in your training runs, if you do take on a carbohydrate gel or sports drink during the race, you will feel like a million dollars!

One of the myths or mistakes critics (often people who have not studied it) make when discussing the ketogenic diet is to assume that it is the "*no*-carb" diet.

This is false—it is a *low*-carb diet. And, in fact, low carb is relative. So if you do no exercise, you may actually need less carbohydrate than someone who trains 4 hours a day. There are many athletes who can eat 150g a day and remain in ketosis—but this will not be everyone.

Dr. Jeff Volek[72] ran the FASTER study (Fat-Adapted-Substrate oxidation in-Trained-Elite-Runners). Zach Bitter was one of the invited participants. The study looked at discovering the role diet plays in how our bodies metabolize fat vs. carbohydrate during exercise.

One portion of the study was a VO2 Max (maximal oxygen uptake) treadmill test. VO2 Max is a partially determining factor in an athlete's aerobic endurance.

During the test, the researchers gradually increased both the speed and incline on the treadmill until the participants could no longer continue and measured rates of fat and carbohydrate metabolism at various intensities.

Zach's fat metabolism peaked at 1.57 grams/minute. At this point in the test, his VO2 uptake was at 49.4. By dividing this number by his eventual VO2 Max of 66.1, he could calculate that at 74.4% intensity he burns the most fat. At that intensity, he was burning 98% fat and 2% carbohydrate.

To put this into perspective, 65% of his VO2 Max had him running approximately a 7:15 per mile.

Even when he increased his speed to around 7:00 per mile, he was still burning nearly all fat! Of course, as the intensity moves up these numbers begin to shift a bit, but you would be surprised at how efficient at fat burning one can be, even at increased intensities.

Zach's Results

% VO2 Max	Fat Usage	Carb Usage
75%	98%	2%
84%	76%	24%
96%	23%	77%

Zach's conclusions[71]:

Even when he started reaching some pretty high (for ultrarunning) intensities (80%+ VO2 Max), he was still metabolizing way more fat than carbs. Brilliant!

An athlete cannot replace the amount of calories they are burning quickly enough to expect an outside fuel source to meet their race-day caloric demands. A person may be able to physically consume enough, but their body would simply not be able to process the fuel quickly enough to stay ahead.

This is why the less need you have to fuel your body during a race the better. Not to mention that fuelling can be a hassle, and if it can be minimized, the hassle lessens.

There are a lot of other factors that come into play as well. Heat, for example, can greatly affect how the body accepts (or, on super-hot days, rejects) the calories you give it. This is why you see so many more stomachs turn at hot weather races. Less eating means your body can use its precious blood stores for cooling and muscle function rather than for digestion.

Are Supplements Essential On The Ketogenic Diet Or Are They Just Marketing Hype?

As mentioned earlier, some people experience the "keto flu" when first starting on the ketogenic diet. They feel tired and irritable. Some of this is normal when simply coming off a sugar addiction. This will pass in a few days. But some of this feeling comes from low electrolyte levels.

When you first start the ketogenic diet, you ingest significantly less sugar. This lowers your blood sugar level so your insulin levels drop as well. As your insulin levels drop, you start to excrete more sodium, potassium and magnesium, therefore it is common to become deficient in these electrolytes in the first few weeks.

If you make a point of topping up these electrolytes initially, you will reduce most of these "keto flu" symptoms immediately.

People who plan ahead and top up their minerals generally do a lot better and tend not to experience "keto flu" symptoms.

Sodium

Normal table salt is not sodium. Table salt is sodium chloride. If you want to top up your sodium, you should take sodium like Himalayan salt.

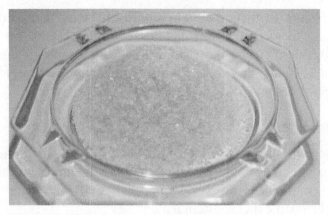

5-7grams of sodium is ideal. Add sodium Himalayan salt to your meals and even to your water.

Potassium

Potassium is widely available in many foods. Eat more potassium-rich foods like spinach and all green leafy vegetables and avocados.

Magnesium

Supplementing with magnesium is good advice for nearly everyone. Most of the population is deficient in magnesium due to poor soil quality that has developed over the years because of modern farming techniques.

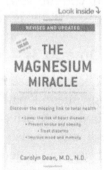

Take magnesium glycerate, which is more easily absorbed than magnesium citrate.

Magnesium has so many benefits. If you want to dive deeper, this book[64], *The Magnesium Miracle*, is excellent.

Many endurance athletes I know swear by adding sodium, magnesium and potassium to their diet. They perform better and recover faster. Incidentally, this applies to athletes both on the ketogenic diet and those not on it. Most people, if tested, would find that they are chronically deficient in electrolytes.

Cartinine

When the body oxidizes a lot of fat, it needs cartinine to transport energy into its cells. The body naturally produces some cartinine. However, it appears that 80-90% people on the ketogenic diet are deficient.

Cartinine is a useful supplement to take.

Vitamin D

Ivor Cummings[65] has done an extensive study on the power of this hormone. Vitamin D deficiency is closely linked with autoimmune disease, cancers, thyroid issues, metabolic syndrome, blood disorders, osteoporosis and heart disease.

Make sure you ask to have your vitamin D levels tested next time you are at the doctors. Most people are deficient—even those in sunny climates.

If you are low, make an effort to get sunshine on a daily basis. If this is not possible, take a supplement.

Omega 3s

These are essential fats vital for your cell health. They are an integral part of cell membranes throughout the entire body and affect the cell receptors in these membranes. Omega-3s also help make hormones that regulate blood, heart, and genetic function.

Studies[66] show that omega 3s help prevent heart disease

and stroke, may help control lupus, eczema, and rheumatoid arthritis, and may protect against cancer.

They are available in plentiful supply in small, cold-water fatty fish such as Wild Planet sardines and mackerel in olive oil and are a great ketogenic food.

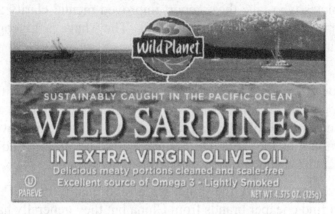

These are far better than any fish oil supplement.

Zinc

Nearly every athlete is deficient in zinc. Zinc is also very difficult to test for. Most nutritionists advise taking a supplement and it is safest to assume you are deficient.

Zinc boosts immunity, helps fight cancer, helps nutritional absorption, helps organ function and aids muscle repair.

Creatine mono-hydrate

There is a definite performance-enhancing effect from creatine. Many athletes take 5g every day. Creatine is the most studied sports nutrition supplement on the market.

There is no disputing its effects. It improves your top end power by around 8%. It is not expensive and works for most people.

Get 8% improvement just by mixing powder into a drink. This is a no-brainer!

Exogenous Ketones

These are much discussed in ketogenic communities. Most athletes who take these report improved mental clarity and improved recovery post workout. They have a glycogen sparing effect.

Dr. Peter Attia[67] has written a great blog post about his experience with exogenous ketones. He discovered that exogenous ketones can actually improve output and stamina for prolonged athletic activity. In fact, there were rumours at the Tour De France that some of the leading riders used supplements with exogenous ketones.

If you want to try these out, get a high quality brand. You can find cheaper brands from China but they generally have added dairy and water.

There are indications that there is less time to exhaustion with exogenous ketones. Should athletes take them? The evidence to date is not conclusive. There are some anecdotally positive results.

More research is being done and more and more products will be coming out to this market as it is potentially huge.

Personally, I do not think you should even consider them until you have done the basics, cleaned up your diet, and really done a solid 12 months on the ketogenic diet.

Understand what it feels like to fuel your body on ketones both at rest and during hard workouts. Make sure you understand (and have implemented!) the fundamentals first before adding ketones.

If you have not fully keto-adapted, adding exogenous

ketones will likely just make you put on weight as you will be adding more fuel that you do not need right now until you are ready.

I have not experimented with exogenous ketones yet. I am dialling in my macro-nutrients. I am taking the mineral supplements as most people are deficient and I already feel a difference with these.

Exogenous ketones I may try after 1 year or so on the ketogenic diet when I am confident I have got the basics covered and have become fat-adapted. I do not want to be adding too many factors at once as it is impossible to know what is working.

Keto Foods

I would also recommend avoiding commercially produced "keto" foods. "Keto" is a trendy term right now and there are a lot of convenience foods being produced with the word "keto" in their descriptions that will not do you any good.

Keep it simple. Eat as many wholesome, natural foods as you can. Ditch the grains, the processed foods and the sugars. Eat more good fats and stay hydrated.

With any change to routine it is easy to read about it and think, *Oh, yes, that makes sense, I will start tomorrow,* and then fall off the wagon in the first 24 hours.

Or you plan enough for the first day then are unable to continue because something trivial threw you off your game.

If you are aware of the common pitfalls, you will enhance your chances of success. Also be aware that, with anything "new" you are trying, you will not be used to it, you need to allow time for adaptation to occur.

So expect your body to protest at first. Your body may like its Mars bars and sugary gels! It won't give them up without a fight ☺

If you are a sugar burner, expect some cravings for the first few days then these will pass. Be prepared for it.

Here are the 7 most common mistakes:

1. Not planning enough

Make sure that, when you start, you plan at least a week's meals in advance. Know what you will eat and when. If you leave it to chance, the likelihood is when you are busy, tired and craving sugar, you will give in very quickly.

If you can get through just one week (not long), you will be fine.

Get rid of the temptations that are around your house like cookies, cakes, breakfast cereal and pastas.

2. Reduced electrolytes

Of course, not everyone gets "keto flu" but if you expect this and take sodium, potassium, magnesium and zinc supplements for the first week, you are more likely to avoid the keto flu and therefore less likely to give up in the first week.

This is an easy win and most people are deficient anyway, so it is likely to give you a boost.

3. Not making meals you enjoy

This should not be difficult. You should not actually feel hungry as you are not restricting calories. Make enjoyable meals with plenty of protein, fat, meats eggs, fish and vegetables.

(In the next chapter, I have provided some typical meals enjoyed by some great endurance athletes so you can get an idea of what they actually eat.)

There is also a plethora of ketogenic recipes available free online so, when you are ready, a simple search will give you an abundance of ideas.

4. Being impatient

Acknowledge that you have eaten one way for many years, decades in fact. It will take some adjustment for a few weeks to get used to eating a different way. Your body will need to adjust, which may take a few weeks.

IT MAY TAKE A FEW DAYS TO A WEEK TO AVOID THE PANGS FOR INSTANT SUGAR

Prepare for it with a strong mind-set but also with healthy food on hand that you can eat without going off the diet.

If you feel like snacking, reach for a handful of nuts or cold meats rather than a handful of cookies.

Remember the Standard American diet (SAD) is 65% carbohydrate. You will be switching from 65% carbs to at least 65% fat. This is a significant change. So be gentle on your body, do not expect instant change and track your results.

If you mess up one meal, or give in to snacking, don't beat yourself up, just start again the next day.

5. Not measuring your carbs

You do not need to count calories but you do need to count your macros initially. It is easy not to know how many carbohydrates are in the food you eat.

If you eat too many carbohydrates, you will not achieve ketosis and you may think the diet does not work. If you are going to try something, make sure you execute it correctly before making a judgement and tossing it out the window too soon.

For example, you may think that nuts are pure protein. However, there is a lot of carbohydrate in cashews and peanuts.

If you want to get into ketosis quickly, aim for 25-50g carbohydrates a day. If this is too difficult initially, you can allow a little more but definitely stay under 100g/day then slowly reduce back down.

You will also go into ketosis faster if you do some aerobic exercise as well. This works even better if you do it in a fasted state.

For example, if you do a workout before breakfast, you are exercising in a fasted state. Your body will be forced to burn fat as there will be very little glucose around.

6. Excessive alcohol

Alcohol is a no-no for those who are trying to do a strict ketogenic diet and lose weight. Apart from adding empty calories, your body can't store alcohol as fat—it has to metabolize it first. As a result, the fat-burning advantage of the ketogenic diet is diminished. Alcohol also increases appetite, causes dehydration and suppresses self-control. None of these work well when you are making a change in routine and diet.

Alcohol converts in your body to acetate and if you are tracking your ketone levels, you will get inaccurate and artificially high results.

7. Too much snacking

Once you have done a couple of weeks on the ketogenic diet, you shouldn't need to snack. This will not involve willpower. The fact is by eating properly you just will not require snacks between meals.

Also be mindful that a lot of extra eating is just due to boredom.

A lot of extra eating is due to procrastination. You don't want to write the paper or clear out the garage so you go make a club sandwich.

And a lot of extra eating is due to unhappiness.

Try to be mindful of this and teach yourself not to eat unless you are actually hungry. Ask yourself if you feel like a snack—is this just a habit or am I hungry?

If you are not hungry, it is fine to skip a meal. This is effectively intermittent fasting, which we discussed earlier.

There is no need to eat just because a man-made item (a clock) is pointing in a certain direction. If you are not hungry, do not eat.

Lack of protein will make you hungry, so make sure you are getting enough. Only snack on real foods not junk.

Look, I'm no chef and I'm not pretending to be. I keep my food simple, quick to prepare and easy. I have given you the list of foods you can and can't eat in chapter 4. But it is super useful to see how these foods fit within actual meals.

This is not going to be a list of pretty recipes for the ketogenic diet. There are already a ton of amazing ketogenic recipes available online that you can access within 2 seconds via a Google search.

Rather than repeat what is already available and creatively presented by awesome chefs, I think there is more value for us to take a sneak peak inside a typical day's eating for real-life endurance athletes who have achieved great success on the ketogenic diet.

Then you can take what they do and replicate it or take what they do and add your own spin with some inspiration from other ketogenic recipes.

If you have eaten the typical Western diet, full of cereals, bread and pastas, it is easy to be completely perplexed and think, *Well, what is there left to eat?*

Keep in mind that you need to tweak this diet for *your needs*. Things that work for someone else will not necessarily work for you.

Also, if you eat exactly what these athletes eat, keep in mind that you may not be training how they train.

In other words, if you are doing sprint triathlons and train 6 hours a week, you should not be eating the same diet (and quantity) as someone who competes in ultra-endurance Ironmans and trains 25 hours a week!

Other considerations include whether you are male or female, body size, current fitness levels, goals, current medications, current state of health, whether you are vegetarian, vegan, diabetic, lactose intolerant, gluten intolerant or have other allergies or illnesses.

The following are examples of what other people do. This does not mean it is what *you* should do. This is for illustration and education purposes only.

Please consult your doctor or nutritionist if you have any medical or health issues. It is recommended that you get your blood work done before starting to get your baseline levels. Then repeat the blood test 4 weeks later so you can measure improvement, learn what is working, get some motivation and highlight any potential issues so you can make adjustments if necessary.

ZACH BITTER

Zach Bitter is one of America's greatest ultra runners. He is the 100 Mile American Record Holder and the 12 Hour World Record Holder.

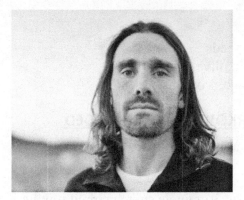

Photo from zachbitter.com

He eats modified ketogenic during the season and is strict ketogenic in the off-season.

This is his typical day[75]:

Pre-Breakfast

Coffee with butter, coconut oil and raw honey
Vespa concentrate

He then trains without food

Run 15 miles
5x 1 mile repeats (5:30/mi) with 1-mile recovery jog between
3 mile cool-down

BREAKFAST

Avocado, sweet potato, carrot, bowl of spinach
Extra virgin olive oil, sea salt
1-cup wild-caught salmon
1 oz. sharp cheddar (preferably raw)
Supplements-vitamin D, Kelp, blue green algae, probiotic, magnesium, coQ10

LUNCH

1 cup flax seeds
Extra virgin olive oil
2 oz. sausage, 1 oz. sharp cheddar

PRE-WORKOUT SNACK IF NEEDED

1-cup raw almonds

Training

7 miles easy, 30-minute stretch/circuit routine

DINNER

Cantaloupe w/ cinnamon
4 oz. fresh calf liver
6 slices bacon
2 cups cabbage, 1 avocado
3 tbsp. sour cream
Turmeric, oregano, sea salt
1 tbsp. butter
Herbal tea with coconut milk and honey

*** ***

SAMI INKINEN

Sami has mastered optimizing physical performance while working 80-90 hour weeks and traveling extensively.

He has two sub 9-hour finishes at the Ironman Hawaii.

Sami was age group world champion at the Half Ironman (70.3.) distance in 2011 and was ranked number #2 age group triathlete in the U.S. in 2009.

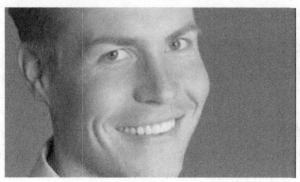

Photo from samiinkinen.com

His fastest Ironman triathlon was 8h24min(2012) and he also had several age group course records at Wildflower and Treasure Island triathlons, as well as 3 consecutive age group wins at the Escape from Alcatraz Triathlon.

During summer 2014, he and his wife rowed across the Pacific Ocean, completely unsupported, from California to Hawaii for 2750 miles. It took 45 days and 3 hours, which is now the speed world record for a two-person crew.

He's an amazing athlete, and it's even more impressive that he has achieved all this whilst running a large company!

This is what he typically eats:

BREAKFAST

500 calories of fat. Coconut butter or coconut oil in coffee It's pretty fast to digest and it doesn't feel like it's in your stomach if you go and work out.

Three to five eggs

LUNCH

Salad with lots of greens and a little bit of protein, so that could be salmon or ground beef and then a lot of olive oil or butter

SNACKS IF NECESSARY

Some sort of meat or sausage or almonds or macadamia nuts

DINNER

A bowl full of sautéed greens with a bunch of butter with some kind of protein. It could be shrimps, fish or beef

He usually drinks water but might have almond milk

*** ***

DR. PETER ATTIA

Dr. Attia is a surgeon, a former McKinsey consultant, and a relentless self-experimenter. He is the president and co-founder of the Nutrition Science Initiative (NuSI). Peter also spent two years at the National Institutes of Health as a surgical oncology fellow at the National Cancer Institute where his research focused on the role of regulatory T cells in cancer regression.

Peter has an excellent blog, The Eating Academy[3], where he explains in great details the biochemistry of the ketogenic diet, his results from his own experiments with the ketogenic diet and athletic performance and how it can apply to the community.

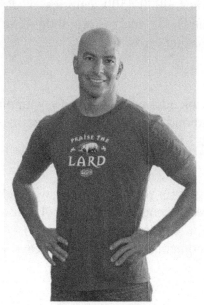

Photo from eatingacademy.com

Dr. Attia earned his M.D. from Stanford University and holds a B.Sc. in mechanical engineering and applied mathematics from Queen's University.

He is also an incredible endurance athlete regularly competing in 25-mile swims and 100+ mile cycling events.

MACROS

Dr. Attia has reduced his carbohydrates from 600g per day (typical American diet) to 50g a day. Keep in mind there is no "right" amount. It depends on your genes and your goals.

The correct protocol will change depending on whether you are doing it for weight loss, athletic performance, to gain energy or for disease reversal.

Peter consumes 4000-4500 calories a day to fuel his athletic demands. His macros are 400g-425g fat, 120-140g protein and 30-50g carbs.

BREAKFAST

Fat shake. In blender add 8oz. heavy whipping cream, 8oz sugar free almond milk, 25m sugar-free hydrolysed whey protein and 2-3 frozen strawberries

Or

Scrambled eggs (6 yolks, 3 whites with added heavy fat cream) cooked in coconut oil, 3 or 4 sausage patties (be sure to look for brands not cured in sugar)
Coffee with homemade whip cream (heavy fat cream hand whipped)

Or

Whole fat latte at Starbucks (made same as above), scrambled eggs, bacon (high fat pieces), slice of Swiss and slice of cheddar

Or

Breakfast: Omelette (6 yolks, 3 whites, coconut milk, sautéed onions) cooked in coconut oil, 4 or 5 pieces of the fattest bacon I can find
2 cups of coffee with heavy cream

LUNCH

Plate of assorted cheeses (aged Gouda, Swiss loaf, aged Parmesan – about 3 oz.), about 2 oz. salami, about 1 oz. olives

Or

Tomatoes with basil and mozzarella and balsamic vinegar and olive oil, about 2 oz. raspberries with homemade whip cream

Or

About 4 oz. of especially fat salami and pepperoni, about 2 oz. Parmesan cheese

Or

Half chicken (thigh, breast, wings) with lots of skin; about 2 oz. of Gouda and aged-cheddar

Or

About 5 oz. of assorted cheese (Gouda, Swiss, Manchego), 2 or 3 oz. olives, about 4 oz. of particularly fat salami and pepperoni

1 cup of decaf coffee with homemade whip cream

DINNER

Garden salad with olive oil (lots of extra oil) and balsamic vinegar dressing, about 6 oz. grilled salmon with a lot of butter and lemon juice

Or

Wedge blue cheese salad with bacon; 12 oz. prime rib with lots of butter; 5 or 6 pieces of asparagus coated in butter

Or

Ground beef sautéed with heavy cream, onions, broccoli, and melted cheese

2 large cups of decaf coffee with homemade whip cream (heavy cream whipped with a touch of xylitol)

Or

Leftover ground beef sautéed from previous night, salad with homemade cream dressing (whole fat Greek yogurt, olive oil, basil, blue cheese, garlic)

1 cup of decaf coffee with homemade whip cream

Or

Cream of mushroom and bacon soup (heavy cream, chicken broth, shredded Parmesan cheese, mushrooms, chopped bacon, garlic, butter, chopped papers, various spices)

Or

Leg of lamb (baked in sauce made of red wine, balsamic vinegar, diced tomatoes, garlic, and a lot of spices)

2 cups decaf coffee with homemade whip cream

SNACKS

About 2 oz. of mixed nuts (almonds, walnuts, peanuts), large latte (made with heavy fat cream instead of milk)

*** ***

As Dr. Attia writes extensively[82] about his ketogenic journey, I have added more depth and explanation of his thoughts behind what he does.

He used to eat a lot of fruits and vegetables and complex carbohydrates, like the iconic athlete's diet where about 65% of his intake was coming from carbohydrates. Now he is really focused on eating a higher quantity of fat.

He is particular about not eating too many omega-6 fats, what he calls "junk oils." He does not really eat many fruits or other vegetables with great regularity besides sautéed onions and mushrooms once in a while, but mostly that's just another way to eat lots of fat, such as butter and coconut oil.

As he exercises a lot, here is a typical Sunday morning:

A five-and-half hour 90 mile (150 km) bike ride at pretty high intensity with 9,000 feet (2,800 m) of climbing.

Before the ride he typically eats bacon, eggs, and heavy cream in his coffee. A ride like that burns about 4,500 calories, but during the ride he will only ingest about 50 grams of something called Superstarch[76] (about 180 calories worth) and about 2 ounces of mixed nuts (approximately 300 to 350 calories).

In other words, he is able to supply his muscles with sufficient energy from existing fat stores and existing glycogen stores, depending on the level of intensity.

When fully loaded, you store about 1,600 calories worth of glycogen. The real point to keep in mind is that it's all about your ability to access your fat stores rather than your glycogen stores.

If you're solely reliant on your glycogen stores, you get into trouble really soon because you're going to deplete those stores. You're going to constantly need to replace glucose during the exercise.

Fat makes up 85-90% of his calories, but this is because he consumes so many calories per day. For many folks in nutritional ketosis, fat makes up 65-75% of their total calories.

Isn't all that fat bad for you?

Dr. Attia says there's not a shred of meaningful scientific evidence to even suggest, let alone demonstrate, that saturated fat is bad for you.

If you're really interested in understanding this topic, a great place to start is reading Gary Taubes' book, *Why We Get Fat*[16], and if you want the more detailed version you should read his other book, *Good Calories, Bad Calories*[17].

In fact, the consumption of simple carbohydrates and sugars is what leads to the presence of elevated triglycerides in your bloodstream, including saturated triglycerides. The same is true for cholesterol. The cholesterol you eat has no bearing on the cholesterol in your bloodstream.

The fat that Dr. Attia does consider bad is omega-6 polyunsaturated fat (e.g., plant oils like soy, canola, sunflower, safflower). The ratio of omega-6 to omega-3 fats one consumes plays a large role in helping mediate inflammation in your body. Therefore he profoundly restricts his intake of omega-6 fats.

STU MITTLEMAN

Stu is the author of *Slow Burn: Burn Fat Faster by Exercising Slower*[70], and a record-setting endurance athlete with degrees in sports psychology and exercise physiology.

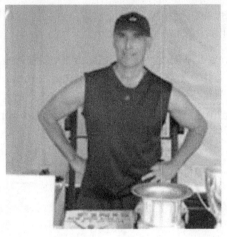

Photo from worldultrafit Facebook page

He has set eight national and international records in long-distance running, including the 1,000-mile world record in 1986. In 2000, he ran across the United States from San Diego to New York—a distance of some 3,000 miles—in 56 days.

He's the current president of WorldUltrafit Inc., his fitness coaching and consulting firm, and a member of motivational speaker and writer Tony Robbins' Mastery University coaching team.

Stu also trained under Dr. Phil Maffetone. Maffetone changed his diet and training approach so that he was using fat as his primary energy source and not sugar.

Stu has the view of keeping it simple. Do not over analyse. Get the basics 80% correct and you will be way ahead of where you were.

He never talks about ketosis or the ketogenic diet. However, from what he eats and discusses, it's clear his philosophy is very similar.

He focuses on eating more fat, significantly reducing sugars and having a little protein.

Stu eats more towards a vegetarian diet (though he has re-introduced fish). He emphasizes salad, spinach, olive oil, garlic and fish. He eats no bread or pasta and selects food high in alkalinizing properties like soy, nuts, green veggies and fish.

HE SAYS (AND I LOVE THIS QUOTE), "FOCUS ON RESULTS AND YOU WON'T CHANGE. FOCUS ON CHANGE AND YOU'LL GET RESULTS."

Stu Mittleman never eats bananas, sports drinks or candy/gels while he is running and instead carries raw almonds, vegetable purees, and avocado with him.

Here are a list of other athletes you may know who also are on the ketogenic diet or doing some form of low carb, high fat regime and getting better results than when they were on a high carb diet.

This list was compiled from a collaboration between Peter Defty—General Manager at Vespa, Optimized Fat Metabolism (OFM)[77]—and Low Carb Down Under[78]

Jon Olsen – previous 100 mile American record holder & 2013 – 24 hour World Champ

Dan Lenz – in 2015 2nd at Umstead 100 miler

Jenny Capel – Winner of San Diego 100 and 4th Overall

Nikki Kimball – Ran the Marathon Des Sables 2014 for the first time and won

Roxanne Woodhouse – at 52 years old won the Zion 100 by almost an hour ahead of Susan Bron a high carb athlete

Mike Morton – in 2013 won both Rocky Raccoon and Iron horse 100 within a week of each other

Jean Pommier – at age 51 2nd Overall in the Ruth Anderson 50 miler

Calum Neff – 2nd at FLS Sugarland 30k a day after winning the Brazos Bend Trail Half Marathon.

Jeremy Humphrey – winner of River of No Return Endurance runs 100km

Bevan Mckinnon – in 2014 won the overall age group race at New Zealand Ironman Triathlon

Bevan[72] has been on a low carb, high fat diet since

November 2013. He has seen excellent results on this diet and is still optimizing it to get greater benefits in metabolic efficiency and fat burning.

His diet is typically three meals a day with protein from animal sources usually along with a very high vegetable intake.

He uses coconut oil, olive oil and butter as his major extra sources of added fat. He avoids industrial seed oils high in Omega 6.

His diet is high in fish, eggs and nuts.

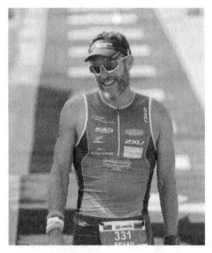

Photo from scientifictriathlon.com

Leading into an Ironman race, Bevan does no special carbohydrate loading or any particular change in diet, apart from some extra kumara (New Zealand version of a sweet potato) in the few meals prior to race.

DINNER THE NIGHT BEFORE AN IRONMAN

Roast pork with crackling, vegetables, kumara

BREAKFAST RACE DAY

Small amount of high fat yogurt, banana, protein powder

Bevan says[79] consumption of carbohydrates for energy produces greater fumes, i.e. a greater amount of CO_2. Fat burns with lower emission of CO_2.

Less CO_2 appears to reduce the build-up of blood lactate, possibly indicating a reduced acidic response within the muscle. From both ventilatory (breathing response) and metabolic (blood lactate) standpoints he finds there is improved economy.

Tim Reed[73] Finished in 1st place in 2015 Ironman 70.3 Auckland- Asia Pacific Championships with the fastest run. He realised he was utterly dependant on carbs to fuel all levels of exercise intensity. He has been making gradual changes towards a low carb, high fat diet since 2010.

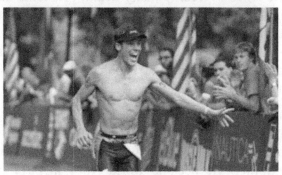

Photo from timreed.com.au

Tim now eats a lot of meat, dairy, eggs, a tonne of vegetables (yes. even carbohydrate-laden root vegies), fruit at the right times, nuts and raw oils.

Instead of thinking about food all the time, he reports that he feels satiated and can go hours before having to run back to the fridge.

Tim Olsen – winner of the 2012 & 2013 Western States 100 mile

The LA Lakers

Members of the Australian Cricket team

Players in major Australian football clubs

There are, of course, many more athletes and sporting teams that are rumoured to be using low carb, high fat strategies to improve performance but are not publicly making it known as they wish to keep one of their competitive advantages secret.

You can't blame them—why would they want to give away one of the key secrets to their dominant success?

One example may be Novak Djokovic.

Djokovic[83] has overcome many health problems that were hindering his performance by banning gluten—which is present in most foods—and dairy products. Early in his career he was forced to take several medical breaks per tournament. He often had trouble breathing, suffered intestinal distress and low physical and mental energy.

Djokovic also cut out as much sugar as possible. He has become arguably the greatest athlete in world tennis, combining stamina and strength with extraordinary speed and flexibility. He became world No 1 in 2011 and has stayed there ever since, apart from a spell to Roger Federer and more recently with Andy Murray.

Djokovic's diet is based on vegetables, beans, white meat, fish, fruit, nuts, seeds, chickpeas, lentils and healthy oils.

He is meticulous about when and how he eats. Djokovic buys organic food wherever possible and cooks almost every meal himself.

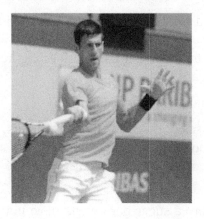

*** ***

How Can You Wean Yourself Off Sports Gels, Chews, and Sugary Sports Drinks?

Let's be clear. This book (and the ketogenic diet) is NOT an anti-carb rant! Carbohydrates are useful when used correctly. The problem is, due to misinformation and marketing, most people have an *over-reliance* on carbohydrate.

The whole point of the ketogenic diet is to stabilize the blood sugar levels, reduce insulin spikes, eat more wholesome, natural foods, less processed junk food in wrappers, and to be able to access our massive resource of fat for unlimited energy instead of having to rely on external sources of energy during a race.

We are seeking improved performance, improved health and mental clarity in both life and sport.

So Should We Ditch The Sports Gels Immediately And Go Cold Turkey?

You can achieve ketosis within 24 hours. But you will not

be fat-adapted for at least 6-12 weeks as the body needs to develop fat-burning pathways, increase its amount of fat-burning enzymes and get used to burning ketones for fuel instead of sugars.

It is best to make gradual changes.

That being said, I see a lot of runners, cyclists and triathletes who take excessive sports drinks and gels when they do not need them at all (even if they are not fat-adapted).

Even if you are a sugar burner and have not fat-adapted at your normal training pace, you still have enough glucose supplies for 2 hours of exercise without bonking.

THERE IS *NO NEED* TO TAKE ON ANY EXTRA CARBOHYDRATE GELS OR DRINKS IF YOUR TRAINING SESSION IS UNDER 2 HOURS

It just gives you unnecessary insulin spikes, extra calories you do not need and feeds a sugar addiction. Plain water is all you need for this training duration.

Plus you are likely to put on body weight over your training time rather than shed excess weight if you take gels every time you step out of the house.

I see some people training for a 5km race and they have had 2 gels and a sports drink during a 30-40 minute jog and wonder why they are not losing weight.

The same holds true for marathon training. Many participants do not lose weight and even put on weight over their training period. For any run under 2 hours, you do NOT require sugary supplements.

Review your own fuelling habits and, whether or not you choose to embrace the ketogenic diet, do make a decision to cut out the extra sugar immediately and your performance will improve.

No one needs it. It will just make you fatter and slower over time.

For any training over 2 hours, if you are not fat-adapted, you will start to feel the lack of energy creep in and will need to top up your glucose levels.

If you decide to implement the ketogenic diet, it will take you several weeks to get fat-adapted so experiment over the weeks. You won't be able to go "cold-turkey" day 1, so take along some gels or sports drink as reserves then see what happens.

Make gradual changes. If you normally take 4 gels on a 3-hour bike ride, aim to take 3 gels then reduce to 2 as you are able. A few weeks later, you should be able to get down to one gel or even none.

Everyone will progress at different rates and will have different metabolisms so you will need to test and measure then make adjustments. Experiment with different fuel like a handful of almonds and see how you go.

Be careful to record your progress in your training diary and gradually take less and less extra sugar on board.

Sometimes taking extra sugar on board is just bad habit, boredom or feeling "tired" so we think a sugar kick might help.

Dr. Jeff Volek's[2] research is showing that ketogenic athletes recover faster and suffer less oxidative stress.

Most of all, be aware of what you are consuming and why. Do not mindlessly take 3 gels an hour just because they are there. It is not doing any favors for your athletic ability, your waistline or your health.

Remember, if your training session or race is >6 hours or longer, it is fine to have some carbohydrates on hand if you need them. However, reduce your reliance on taking them for *every* training session.

If you keep taking on sugar, you will never give your body a chance to unlock the abundant energy contained in your fat stores.

Carbohydrates have their place. There is no denying they work. Just make sure you are their master not their slave.

As with ANY diet, there is no "one size fits all". There is only looking at what works for other people, testing it out and seeing if it works for you.

Equally, it is true that people succeed on vastly different diets. Michael Arnstein[80] (one of the best 100 mile runners in USA) eats nothing but fruit (literally—he is a fruitarian!) and runs 30 miles a day. He finished 29th in the New York Marathon in 2011.

Some people succeed on heavy meat diets; some people succeed on totally plant-based diets; others prefer a bit of both.

Be clear about your goals and why you wish to address your diet.

Is it to lose weight ASAP?
Is it to improve your athletic performance in the next year or two?
Is it to have enhanced athletic performance plus long-term health and longevity?

All of these will result in a different emphasis for your diet.

The mistake many people make is there are "so many diets" out there; they try to research them all, become experts on all of them trying to find the Holy Grail that is the best diet.

It is easy to get very confused and go down so many different rabbit holes that you never end up making a start on any of them.

I suggest just picking one and doing that for 6 months. Track your food intake, your metrics—BMI, weight, body fat%—plus your training results and how you feel.

Then tweak it or change it later on if you find it does not suit you.

But the quickest way to get change is to start now!

The most common element of all diets is to cut out take-aways, fast food and artificial products in wrappers filled with chemicals and preservatives. Try as best you can to eat natural foods.

Whilst there are pros and cons of any way of eating, I believe keeping it as simple as possible is by far the best way of eating that you can fit in to your day, that does not make you miserable, that makes sense to you and that you can sustain.

Your body is metabolically flexible enough to be able to switch between using fat and glucose for energy with little or no drop in performance.

Fat-adaption involves nutritional ketosis and carbohydrates may be used strategically throughout training and racing to enhance performance.

Review Your Diet

Get the fundamentals right.

If you are not the body shape you desire, or not getting the athletic results you think you deserve, diet is often a huge factor that athletes neglect.

It is not enough to say, "I train so much that I can get away with eating junk food." Sure, you will likely be "fine" for a year or two. But junk food will not yield you the best performance results you are capable of. Plus you do not want to be a sitting time bomb for chronic disease down the track.

One thing is for sure, doing the same thing in the future as you did in the past will not change your results.

From my research, I feel the ketogenic diet makes sense for most individuals from a health point of view and athletic performance reasons. It is not a new fad diet. It has been scientifically validated since the 1920s with proven results treating epilepsy.

There is a lot of research (and amazing anecdotal evidence) currently going on with athletic performance plus in treating other chronic illness like diabetes, cancers and heart disease with the ketogenic diet, which is very exciting.

Quite simply, it is clear that the current way of eating is causing huge problems and disease epidemics throughout the Western world and any cultures who also adopt the Western diet start to see similar issues.

Decide:

You may choose to move slowly towards a ketogenic diet and get your carbs below 150g/day
or
You may be more extreme and restrict carbs below 50g a day
or
You may choose to do a ketogenic diet part of the year and cycle in and out of it

If you decide to make a significant change, do keep a journal of what you are eating and how you are feeling. It is very hard to remember the details a few months down the track.

It is also sensible to check in with your doctor before you start. Get your baseline blood work done to see how you are in terms of cholesterol, blood sugars, blood lipids, vitamins and minerals.

Then start your program and get these tests done again in one month's time.

This will either give you immense motivation in knowing that you are on the right track or may highlight potential issues before they become a problem.

If you are ill or taking regular medication, definitely consult with your doctor before starting this type of radical change.

Review Your Training

Remember to consider the way you train.

If you do 90% anaerobic, you may not be getting the best results you are capable of.

If you do 90% "no man's land" training, you definitely won't be getting the results you are capable of and you may be storing some health issues for later on.

Consider really understanding and implementing periodization of training blocks.

Consider doing 8 weeks base training every year no matter how fit you already are.

Consider adding in more rest if you feel over trained, get sick often or feel constantly stressed.

Even as an experiment try the MAF test and see if you can do your normal "easy workout" at 180-your age beats per minute. You may be surprised how difficult this is.

I was shocked. I am fit and have been fit my whole life. I have trained at a high level most of this time. I thought I would jog slowly round the oval 10 times below my MAF test heart rate.

No way!

I could not even jog slowly one lap without my heart rate shooting up. I had to jog 10 steps, walk 30 steps, jog 10 steps, and walk 30 steps in order to keep my heart rate down to the right level.

Let me tell you, it was an exercise in humility!

Anyway, I made the decision to persist with it and have now improved 25% in just 5 weeks. I am now able to jog most of the laps round the oval below the MAF heart rate (though there is still a little bit of walking in there, it is much reduced).

I will continue to be strict with my aerobic training and continue to improve the speed I can run at my aerobic heart rate. I am excited about the results and can't wait for racing season to start again.

*** ***

Over To You

I do hope you enjoyed this book and it provided you food for thought and some good training ideas. I believe it makes a lot of sense and is worthwhile trying for you.

If you enjoyed this book or received value from it in any way then I'd like to ask you for a favor: would you be kind enough to leave a review for this book on Amazon? I would be so grateful.

Click here to leave a review on Amazon.com or Amazon.co.uk

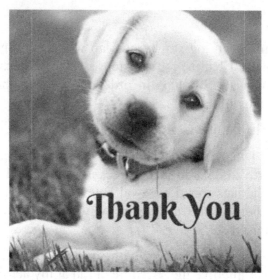

I have provided a ton of resources for you in the next section if you wish to dive deeper and do more research.

This topic is of increasing interest to the scientific, medical and athletic communities. There will be enormous applications to athletic performance and disease prevention and treatment.

Also there is a ton of money going into research for ketone esters and exogenous ketones. I will be watching this space closely and when the science becomes more consistent and there is more widespread use of them, I may decide to experiment with them a little and will report back to you.

I would love to know your thoughts and your experiences.

By the way, if you are a triathlete or are thinking of trying a triathlon, you are welcome to join our Free 5-Day Triathlon Accelerator Course (http://www.triathlon-hacks.com/free-course)

Please feel free to let me know your thoughts.

You can contact me here

Charlotte1@triathlon-hacks.com

Also let me know if you have tried the ketogenic diet and had either positive or negative experiences with it.

Happy training and good luck,

Charlotte

Charlotte
charlotte1@triathlon-hacks.com

Here are the references and resources you may find useful for further reading:

1. Stephen D Phinney and Jeff S Volek The Art and Science of Low Carbohydrate Living: An Expert Guide to Making the Life-Saving Benefits of Carbohydrate Restriction Sustainable and Enjoyable (2011)

2. Stephen D Phinney and Jeff S Volek The Art and Science of Low Carbohydrate Performance (2012)

3. http://eatingacademy.com/nutrition/the-interplay-of-exercise-and-ketosis-part-ii

4. http://firstendurance.com/modified-ketogenic-diet-for-endurance-athletes/

5. http://bayesianbodybuilding.com/ketogains-menno-henselmans/

6. http://www.ncbi.nlm.nih.gov/pubmed/15640462

7. https://www.ncbi.nlm.nih.gov/pubmed/1548337

8. https://www.ncbi.nlm.nih.gov/pmc/articles/PMC3106288/

9. https://www.ncbi.nlm.nih.gov/pubmed/24048020

10. https://www.reddit.com/r/keto/

11. http://180nutrition.com.au/180-tv/this-may-shock-you-what-the-experts-eat-with-world-class-ironman-sami-inkinen/

12. https://philmaffetone.com/180-formula/

13. http://zachbitter.com/blog/

14. https://philmaffetone.com/method/

15. http://www.vespapower.com/

16. Gary Taubes Why We Get Fat and What To Do About It (2012)

17. Gary Taubes Good Calories, Bad Calories:Fats, Carbs, and the Controversial Science of Diet and Health (2008)

18. Tim Noakes. The Lore of Running (2001) First published 1985

19. http://www.health24.com/Diet-and-nutrition/Nutrition-basics/Tim-Noakes-on-carbohydrates-20120721

20. Professor Tim Noakes, Jonno Proudfoot and Sally-Ann Creed. The Real Meal Revolution: The Radical, Sustainable Approach to Healthy Eating (2015)

21. http://realmealrevolution.com/real-thinking/ketosis

22. https://www.ncbi.nlm.nih.gov/pmc/articles/PMC1325029/

23. https://authoritynutrition.com/ketogenic-diet-to-fight-cancer/

24. https://www.ncbi.nlm.nih.gov/pmc/articles/PMC4215472/

25. http://www.ncbi.nlm.nih.gov/pubmed/26782788

26. http://www.epilepsy.com/learn/treating-seizures-and-epilepsy/dietary-therapies/ketogenic-diet

27. https://www.diabetescare.abbott/precision-xtra.html

28. https://storefront.novacares.com/storefront/nova-max-plus-meter.html

29. http://eatingacademy.com/nutrition/welcome-to-the-war-on-insulin

30. https://en.wikipedia.org/wiki/John_Yudkin

31. https://www.youtube.com/watch?v=dBnniua6-oM

32. http://www.nytimes.com/2002/07/07/magazine/what-if-it-s-all-been-a-big-fat-lie.html

33. http://www.runnersworld.com/ask-the-coaches/ask-the-coaches-rectal-bleeding

34. http://ketogains.com/2015/10/the-art-and-science-of-low-carbohydrate-performance-by-jeff-s-volek-and-stephen-d-phinney-a-summary/

35. http://firstendurance.com/ketogenic-diet-for-endurance-performance-should-i-try-it-out/

36. Mark Sisson. Primal Endurance. Escape chronic cardio and carbohydrate dependency and become a fat-burning beast! (2016)

37. http://zachbitter.com/blog/

38. https://www.ncbi.nlm.nih.gov/pmc/articles/PMC2495396/pdf/postmedj00315-0056.pdf

39. http://www.ncbi.nlm.nih.gov/pubmed/24068332

40. https://www.myhealthwire.com/news/breakthroughs/895

41. http://www.leangains.com

42. https://www.ncbi.nlm.nih.gov/pmc/articles/PMC2622429/

43. https://www.ncbi.nlm.nih.gov/pubmed/21106691

44. http://www.translationalres.com/article/S1931-5244(14)00200-X/abstract?cc=y=

45. http://www.ncbi.nlm.nih.gov/pubmed/15640462

46. https://www.ncbi.nlm.nih.gov/pubmed/2355952

47. https://www.ncbi.nlm.nih.gov/pubmed/17291990/

48. http://zachbitter.com/blog/2014/04/intermittent-fasting-feast-or-famine-for-endurance-athletes.html

49. http://www.precisionnutrition.com/intermittent-fasting/summary

50. http://www.triathlon-hacks.com/ironman-triathlon-training/

51. https://www.youtube.com/watch?v=Y6U728AZnV0

52. http://rw.runnersworld.com/selects/pure-heart.html

53. http://www.slowtwitch.com/News/Steve_Larsen_gone_at_39_816.html

54. http://www.xtri.com/all-articles/detail/284-itemId.511706698.html

55. http://www.bodyandsoul.com.au/mind-body/wellbeing/real-life-how-a-heart-attack-changed-my-life/news-story/cae92523c8887f80697a66f3c88a7735

56. http://www.triathlon-hacks.com/heart-rate-variability-training/

57. https://philmaffetone.com/

58. http://www.triathlon-hacks.com/strength-training-triathletes/

59. https://philmaffetone.com/180-formula/

60. https://philmaffetone.com/maf-test/

61. http://www.artandscienceoflowcarb.com/research/

62. http://www.samiinkinen.com/post/11347268687/hawaii-ironman-secrets

63. https://www.outsideonline.com/1920971/brian-mackenzies-controversial-new-approach-marathon-training

64. Carolyn Dean The Magnesium Miracle. Revised and Updated (2014) First published 2007

65. https://www.youtube.com/watch?v=x3hZ9P8GmLs

66. http://www.hsph.harvard.edu/nutritionsource/omega-3-fats/

67. http://eatingacademy.com/personal/experience-exogenous-ketones

68. https://run.mcmillanrunning.com/the-marathon-long-

run/

69. http://www.marksdailyapple.com/health-benefits-of-intermittent-fasting/

70. https://www.amazon.com/Slow-Burn-Faster-Exercising-Slower/dp/0062736744

71. http://zachbitter.com/blog/2014/04/takeaways-from-the-faster-study.html

72. https://lowcarbdownunder.com.au/fats-vs-carbs-what-do-the-elites-know-that-we-dont/

73. http://www.triathlonmag.com.au/nutrition/7683-tim-reed-low-carb-diet-key-to-marathon-703-racing

74. https://profgrant.com/2014/03/04/how-to-win-the-ironman-on-lchf/

75. http://zachbitter.com/blog/2013/03/evolving-diet-and-sample-day.html

76. https://www.generationucan.com/super.html

77. http://www.vespapower.com/ofm/what-is-ofm/

78. https://lowcarbdownunder.com.au/

79. http://www.fitter.co.nz/

80. http://www.thefruitarian.com/

81. Simopoulos, Artemis P. (2008). "The Importance of the Omega-6/Omega-3 Fatty Acid Ratio in Cardiovascular Disease and Other Chronic Diseases". *Experimental Biology and Medicine*. 233 (6): 674–88. doi:10.3181/0711-MR-311. PMID 18408140.

82. https://asweetlife.org/the-ketogenic-diet-and-peter-attias-war-on-insulin/

83. http://www.independent.co.uk/sport/tennis/revealed-the-diet-that-saved-novak-djokovic-8775333.html

Made in the USA
Las Vegas, NV
01 June 2024

90620189R00079